NEUROSCIENCE

Edited by **Thomas Heinbockel**

Neuroscience
Edited by Thomas Heinbockel

Published by InTech
Janeza Trdine 9, 51000 Rijeka, Croatia

Publishing Process Manager Ivona Lovric

Technical Editor Teodora Smiljanic

Cover Designer InTech Design Team

Additional hard copies can be obtained from orders@intechopen.com

Neuroscience, Edited by Thomas Heinbockel
p. cm.
ISBN 978-953-51-0617-3

For EU product safety concerns:
IN TECH d.o.o., Prolaz Marije Krucifikse Kozulić 3, 51000 Rijeka, Croatia,
info@intechopen.com or visit our website at intechopen.com.

Meet the editor

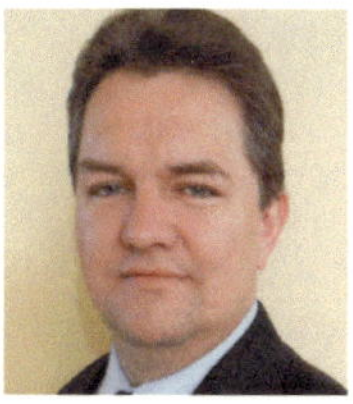

Dr Thomas Heinbockel, Ph.D., is currently Associate Professor, Director of Graduate Studies, and Interim Chairman in the Department of Anatomy, Howard University College of Medicine, Washington, DC, USA. Dr Heinbockel studied biology at the Philipps-University, Marburg, Germany. His studies of the brain started during his M.S. thesis work at the Max-Planck-Institute for Behavioral Physiology, Starnberg/Seewiesen, Germany. Subsequently, he completed a Ph.D. in Neuroscience at the University of Arizona, Tucson, Arizona, USA. After graduating, he held a Research Associate position at the Institute of Physiology, Otto-von-Guericke-University School of Medicine, Magdeburg, Germany. Prior to his arrival at Howard University, Dr Heinbockel held joint research faculty appointments in the Department of Anatomy & Neurobiology and the Department of Physiology at the University of Maryland School of Medicine, Baltimore, Maryland, USA.

Contents

Preface

If one asks what neuroscience is, the answer can be found in this book. Neuroscience embraces not only anatomical and physiological studies but also cell biology, computer science, and biochemistry. Equally important for neuroscientific research are other disciplines, such as psychology, psychiatry, neurology and additional recent ones, such as neuroeconomics and social neuroscience. This book comprises chapters on diverse topics in neuroscience ranging from cellular, computational, cognitive, and clinical neuroscience. Individual chapters focus on recent advances in specific areas including social neuroscience, which is a relatively new field that studies the neural basis of social interactions. Other chapters focus on technological developments such as optical tools to study the function of the brain. All chapters represent recent contributions to the rapidly developing field of neuroscience and illustrate the range of research conducted under the umbrella of the truly interdisciplinary neurosciences. Therefore, this book epitomizes brain research broadly at this particular moment in the evolution of the field. By covering different interdisciplinary topics, this book aims at helping to overcome the department and discipline silos that hold back our research progress in favor of collaborative research teams that engage in successful collaborations to ask questions about the structure and function of the brain and nervous system.

The book is organized into three somewhat overlapping sections: I. Cellular & Computational Neuroscience, II. Cognitive & Social Neuroscience, and III. Clinical & Cognitive Neuroscience. These sections reflect a diverse range of topics covered in the book and at the same time represent major topics in modern neuroscience.

The book begins with a chapter about basic mechanisms of information processing in the brain employed by its constituents, the neurons. Neurons are complex operating devices that use action potentials to encode information. Action potentials are not as static as previously thought and, therefore, Partsvania and Sulaberidze (chapter 1) ask the question 'Is the action potential waveform constant?'

In chapter 2, 'Electrophysiological Recording and Imaging of Neuronal Signals in Brain Slices', Heinbockel describes experiments that test the effects of two pivotal neurotransmitter systems and their relevance for neural network activity: metabotropic glutamate receptors and cannabinoid receptors. Neurons release glutamate as a well-known neurotransmitter and they also release endogenously produced cannabinoids (endocannabinoids) as a retrograde signaling molecule. The effects of endocannabinoids on neurons are mimicked by their exogenous counterpart (tetrahydrocannabinol) found in marijuana (cannabis). Various experimental techniques come into play in this chapter ranging from electrophysiological techniques (patch-clamp recording in brain slices), gene knockout technology (transgenic mice), optical tools (laser flash photolysis, confocal microscopy), and neural staining techniques.

In chapter 3, 'Neuropsychological context of marital functioning', Rostowski and Rostowska address the relationship of brain function and social behavior, specifically marriage. The chapter provides a refreshing look at 'Interpersonal Neurobiology', emphasizing the relevance of the connection of interpersonal relationships, emotions and the brain. The authors elaborate on the system of mirror neurons that influence close social behaviors.

In chapter 4, 'Apraxia: clinical types, theoretical models, and evaluation', Osiurak and Le Gall provide a framework that allows the assessment of disorders which are generally viewed as apraxia. Traditionally, apraxia has been defined as a disorder of skilled movement without attributing it to elementary sensorimotor deficit, aphasia or severe mental deterioration. The authors take the reader to the discovery of apraxia and all the way back to recent proposals regarding its classification and evaluation.

In chapter 5, 'Neurocognitive deficits in patients with Obstructive Sleep Apnea Syndrome (OSAS)', Andreou, Vlachos and Makanikas address a problem in cognitive and clinical neuroscience, namely, Obstructive Sleep Apnea Syndrome (OSAS). The authors describe this sleep disorder and its relation to neurological and cognitive deficits. The authors also review the literature on possible treatment options as well as the neuroanatomical substrates and pathophysiological manifestations of OSAS.

In chapter 6, 'Cognitive disturbances in Sneddon and Antiphospholipid Syndromes',

Rahmani, El Alaoui Faris, Benabdeljlil, and Aidi report on another topic in cognitive and clinical neuroscience, namely, the relationship of a specific type of skin disease (generalised livedo racemosa of the skin) and recurrent stroke. The authors discuss the question whether Sneddon's syndrome overlaps with primary antiphospholipid antibody syndrome (APS) and systematic lupus erythromatosis (SLE).

In chapter 7, 'Cognitive features of vascular dementia', Kwon reviews the relationship of cerebrovascular disease and dementia. The author raises a critical issue, namely, the early accurate diagnosis which is so crucial to the effective management of patients with vascular dementia. Kwon states that recognition of a specific pattern of neuropsychological impairment could be a good diagnostic tool of vascular dementia. Different forms of vascular dementia exist, each with a specific time course of the clinical manifestation of dementia.

Having completed this book, I am grateful to InTech – Open Access Publisher for initiating this book project and for asking me to serve as its editor. Many thanks go to Ms Ivona Lovric at InTech for guiding me through the publication process and for moving the book ahead in a timely fashion. Thanks are due to all contributors of this book for taking the time to first write a chapter proposal, compose their chapter and, lastly, make requested revisions to it. Hopefully, all contributors will continue their neuroscience research with many intellectual challenges and exciting new directions. I would like to thank my wife Dr. Vonnie D.C. Shields, Professor, Towson University, Towson, MD and our son Torben Heinbockel for allowing me to spend time on this book project during the past year. Finally, I am grateful to my parents Erich and Renate Heinbockel for their support over many years.

Thomas Heinbockel, Ph.D.
Associate Professor and Interim Chairman,
Department of Anatomy,
Howard University College of Medicine, Washington, DC,
USA

Section 1

Cellular and Computational Neuroscience

1

Is the Action Potential Waveform Constant?

Besarion Partsvania and Tamaz Sulaberidze
Vladimer Chavchanidze Institute of Cybernetics of the Georgian Technical University, Georgia

1. Introduction

Neurons perform multiple operations. These operations include the receiving of information, processing, coding and transmitting it to other neurons. These involve synapses, membrane ionic channels and changes in membrane potential. The operations are thought of as steps in an algorithm or as computations. The concept of a neuron as a simple integrator unit is antiquated. A neuron could be regarded as complex processor with mixed analogue-digital logic and highly adaptive synaptic elements. Individual nerve cells convert the incoming streams of binary pulses into analogue, spatially distributed variables, such as postsynaptic membrane potential and calcium distribution throughout the dendritic tree and cell body. A number of transformations are applied to these variables which might be understood as subtraction and addition, low- and band-pass filtering, normalization, etc. (Koch, 1999).

"The mammalian brain contains more than 10^{10} densely packed neurons that are connected to an intricate network. In every small volume of the cortex, thousands of spikes are emitted each millisecond. For a long time it has been thought that most of the relevant information was contained in the mean firing rate of the neuron. The firing rate was defined by a temporal average. The concept of mean firing rates has been successfully applied during the last 80 years. It is clear, however, that an approach based on a temporal average neglects all of the information that might be contained in the exact timing of the spikes. From behavioural experiments, it is known that reaction times are often short. Temporal averaging can work well in cases where the stimulus is constant or slowly varying and does not require a fast reaction from the organism. Real inputs change on a fast time-scale. A fly can react to new stimuli and change the direction of flight within 30-40 ms; it has to respond after a postsynaptic neuron has received one or two spikes. Humans can recognize visual scenes in just a few hundred milliseconds. This does not leave enough time to perform temporal averages on each level. In fact, humans can detect images in a sequence of unrelated pictures even if each image is shown for only 14-100 milliseconds. In some cases, a neuron might be driven by an external stimulus which is suddenly switched. For example, when we look at a picture, our gaze jumps from one point to the next. After each saccade, the photo receptors in the retina receive a new visual input. Information about the onset of a saccade would easily be available in the brain and it could serve as an internal reference signal. In such a scenario, it is possible that there exists a code where, for each neuron, the timing of the *first* spike after the reference signal contains all of the information about the new stimulus. In such cases, each neuron transmits exactly one spike per stimulus and it is clear that only the timing conveys information rather than the number of spikes. In the hippocampus, in the olfactory system, and also in other areas of the brain, oscillations of some global variable (e.g., the population activity) are quite common. These oscillations could serve as an internal reference signal. Neuronal spike trains could then encode information in the phase of a pulse with respect to the background oscillation. There is, for example, evidence that the phase of a spike during an oscillation in the hippocampus of rats conveys information on the spatial location of the animal which is not fully accounted for by the firing rate of the neuron" (Gerstner & Kistler, 2002).

The next step in information coding was "rate codes" (Tateno & Robinson, 2006). In fact, there are three different notions of rate, the three definitions of which refer to three different averaging procedures: either an average over time, an average over several repetitions of the experiment, or an average over a population of neurons.

In the view of the above mentioned codes, an action potential (AP) is normalized into a stereotypical form. However, recently we have witnessed another approach to information processing in the single neuron. An ongoing debate surrounds the question of the temporal resolution at which information is represented by individual APs. The longstanding view that an AP is an unchangeable thing has now been challenged.

There is a method of neuron stimulation called "conductance injection" (or "dynamic clamp") (Robinson, 1994). Conductance - representing the response to patterns of presynaptic firing - is applied to the neuron such that current is injected according to the instantaneous value of this conductance and the neuron's membrane potential. Conductance injection reproduces the current-limiting and shunting behaviour and the other dynamical aspects of real synaptic inputs. If experiments are done using conductance injection, the shapes of the resulting APs follow a characteristic width–height distribution. With this method it is possible to look up its immediate conductance history for each spike. The conductance histories leading to different AP waveforms are different: higher background conductance results in broader spikes.

In a study by de Polavieja et al. (2005), dynamic conductance stimulus patterns were used to investigate whether spike shapes reliably depend on the previous stimulus history. They show that in cortical neurons AP waveforms depend on the previous 50 ms of the conductance stimulus history. The authors concluded that this relationship is low in noise, carrying three to four times more information than spike times alone. Although spike frequency and spike shape are related, in general, it is only the spike shape which reliably depends on the different features of the stimulus history on a trial-by-trial basis.

It was shown by Koch & Segev (2000) that for a spike rate of 10 AP/sec, a code based on AP waveforms can transmit 200 bits/sec, compared to the 50 bits/sec of a code based on spike times. It becomes clear that the interaction between incoming postsynaptic potentials and a back propagating AP - as well as, therefore, the probability of producing the next spike - depends upon the AP waveform.

In a recent work, Juusola et al. (2007) have shown that the different AP shapes produced by the same pyramidal cortical neuron are not random but correspond to the level of the previous conductance. The authors named this phenomenon the "AP waveform code". It is proposed that the code influences postsynaptic targets in different ways. One of these ways sees APs of different shapes interacting with incoming excitatory postsynaptic potentials (EPSPs) and influencing synaptic integration differently. Another way could be that the variability of AP waveforms might be saved in the synaptic terminal until a different calcium influx translates these variables into different EPSP sizes in the postsynaptic cell.

Shu et al. (2006) have shown that the somatic AP waveforms survive axonal conduction. It was also shown that the differences in the somatic AP waveforms are further augmented by axonal conduction. This result was obtained using simultaneous somatic and axonal recordings. Furthermore, the EPSPs that they recorded were larger when the presynaptic somatic and axonal spikes were broader.

Häusser et al. (2001) have shown that because the cortical APs of different waveforms differentially shunt incoming synaptic events, they participate in the synaptic integration and the generation of succeeding APs. Therefore, at least 50 ms of the stimulus history can affect the state of the synaptic integration of the neuron and the generation of spikes, through the modulation of the waveform. This is a form of local encoding at the single-neuron level with a 50-ms-long memory, which affects neuronal communication by influencing the production of future spikes.

In summary, for a long time it was thought that the waveform of the AP was constant. However, new evidence continues to show the opposite: it has become clear that the waveform of an AP carries information.

The question arises: Is it possible that the AP waveform contains information about habituation when a single neuron is stimulated with intracellular current impulses and habituates to the stimulation?

The most desirable experiment for answering this question might consider conductance injection into the single neuron. However, there are major limitations to conductance injection. It has to be fast and temporally consistent. For this reason, we decided to stimulate a single neuron with the injection of short current impulses and investigate habituation to the stimulation. We investigated the possible relation of changes of the AP's parameters (and consequently the AP waveform) with the process of habituation.

2. Materials and methods

The isolated nervous system of the mollusc *Helix pomatia* was used in the experiments. Each snail was anesthetized by the injection of isotonic $MgCl_2$, described elsewhere (Patsvania et al., 2008). Then the nervous system was separated from the body. Ganglia were treated with 0.5% Pronaze solution (Protease from Streptomyces griseus - "Sigma-Aldrich") for 30 minutes at room temperature. After proteolytic treatment, the conjunctive tissue was carefully removed using fine micro scissors. Then, the ganglia were washed several times with Ringer solution. This solution consists of: NaCl - 80 mmol, KCl - 4 mmol, $CaCl_2$ - 35 mmol, $MgCl_2 .6 H_2O$ - 5 mmol, Tris -7 mmol at pH=7.5. The nervous system was placed in a Petri dish and positioned in a Faraday cage to filter out any environmental electromagnetic noise. The identified giant neuron #3 of the Left Parietal Ganglion was selected for the investigation. The average diameter of this neuron was 150-200 μm. Identifications were made according to Arakelov et al. (1991). The most naturalistic means of stimulating the neuron is through synaptic input. Antidromic excitation of the nerve with direct current (DC) or pulsed voltage causes AP firing in the inter-neurons, which in turn excites the investigated neuron synaptically. However, if voltage is applied at different locations, the nerve reactions will differ from each other. For this reason, with nerve stimulation it is impossible to maintain any invariance of stimulation. This was the reason for which we chose neuron stimulation with intracellular short current impulses. In this case, it is easy to obtain a condition where the neuron reacts with one AP to one intracellular stimulating impulse. On the other hand, the current stimulating impulse has to be much shorter than the latency period in order to avoid the blending of the AP with the stimulating impulse. The reaction of the neuron depends on the amplitude of the intracellular stimulating impulses. Stimulation was always begun with impulses of a very low amplitude. At the beginning of each recording, the critical value of the intracellular stimulating impulse was established which depolarized the neuron to the threshold and caused the firing of an AP. The experiments showed that this value was always above 0.05 nA and varied from neuron to neuron. Each stimulus triggered only one AP. As such, the reaction pattern consisted of one AP as a reaction to one intracellular stimulating impulse. First, we established the value of the threshold (i.e. we found the critical value of the stimulus that depolarised a neuron to the threshold and caused the firing of only one AP). Next, we increased the amplitude of the stimulus to slightly higher than this critical value.

Figure 1 illustrates a neuron reaction to stimulation with intracellular impulses of an increasing amplitude.

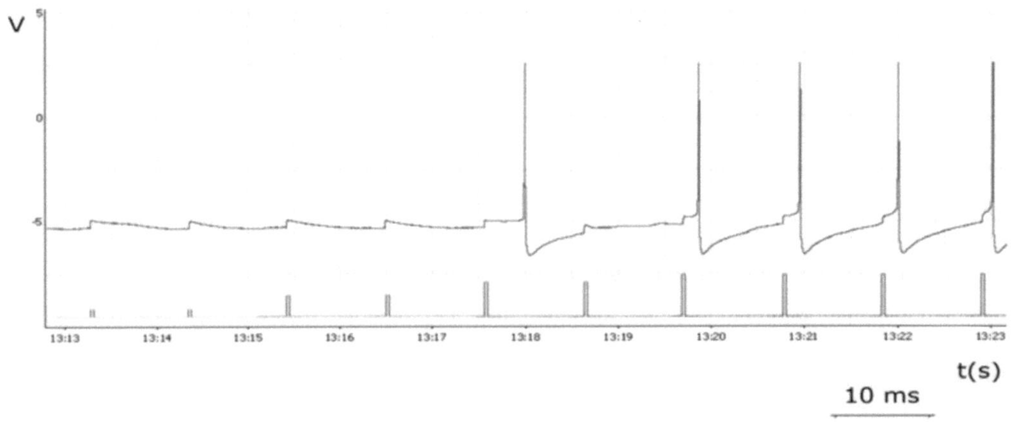

Fig. 1. Neuron reaction to stimulation with increased intracellular current impulses. Current stimulating impulses are shown schematically under the recording. The first four impulses evoke only small shift of membrane potential towards depolarization. The fifth stimulating impulse, with an amplitude 0.5 nA evoked the AP firing of the neuron. The sixth stimulating impulse and those following it have an amplitude of 0.6 nA. The duration of each intracellular impulse is 0.4 ms. It is obvious that this duration is much shorter than the latency period (the latency period is defined as the time interval between the front edge of stimulating impulse and the time moment when membrane potential crosses the threshold value).

For intracellular stimulation, the neuron was impaled with two glass microelectrodes (ME) filled with 2.5 mol KCl. For this purpose, "Piezo Mikromanipulators - PM 20" (Märzhäuser, Wetzlar, Germany) were used. The ME were prepared from capillaries - Borosilicate Tubing (PYREX©) BF 150 75 10 - with filaments (Sutter Instrument Company, Novato, CA, USA). The size of the microelectrode tip was less than 1 μm. The resistance of each microelectrode did not exceed 15 mOhm. Microelectrodes were connected to the "intracellular electrometer IE 251A" (Warner Instruments). One microelectrode served for registration and the other for intracellular stimulation. "Picoamper source K 261" (Keithley Instruments Inc., Cleveland, OH, USA) was used for intracellular stimulation. The output of this device was controlled by a specially designed pulse breaker guaranteeing the application of depolarizing current impulses to the neuron. The intracellular stimuli consisted of a train of depolarizing current impulses, each with a 4 ms width. The frequency of these impulses was 0.9 Hz. This value is close to the frequency of the AP firing of many of the pacemaker neurons of the mollusc ganglion which are synaptically connected to the investigated LPG#3. The PowerLab ML866 data acquisition unit (ADInstruments Co., Castle Hill, NSW, Australia) was used for the registration of experimental data. In Table 1, the variables measured in our experiments are given. All of these variables were measured for each AP. Consequently, sets of numbers were obtained for each experiment. The sets contain data about latent periods, W20s, Tr and Areas. Measurements were performed using the "peak analysis module" for the software "Chart-5".

Parameter description.	Notation
The time interval between the leading edge of the intracellular stimulating impulse and the appearance of AP triggering.	Latency Period
Width of the AP at the level of 20% from the baseline. The baseline corresponds to the neuron resting potential.	W20
Increasing time between two levels (10% and 90 % from the baseline) on the leading edge of the AP.	Tr
Area between the waveform and the baseline.	Area

Table 1. Designations used in the text.

3. Results

Neuron reactions to the intracellular current impulses depend on the amplitude and width of the stimulating impulses. The neuron reacted to the intracellular stimulating impulses with an AP several times, and then habituation arose. Habituation was expressed as a decline of the stimulus-induced AP. The time necessary for habituation varied from several seconds to 1-2 minutes. This time span covers the period between the first intracellular stimulating impulse and the last intracellular impulse after which no more AP was evoked. There is a one-to-one relationship between the time of habituation and the number of APs (or stimulating impulses). For this reason, we define the time of habituation as the amount of stimulating impulses necessary to give rise to habituation. For the purposes of illustration, a sample of the habituation dynamics for one of the neurons is shown in Figure 2.

After habituation, the recovery of the neuron required 15-20 minutes and a new series of stimulation might trigger APs. However, the new response was shorter and habituation was established sooner. For this reason, each neuron was stimulated with the train of intracellular impulses only once.

The parameters of AP, latent period (and consequently AP waveform) were not constant and varied during stimulation. Figure 3 shows a typical change of AP parameters and latent period evoked by the application of the recurrent intracellular current impulses.

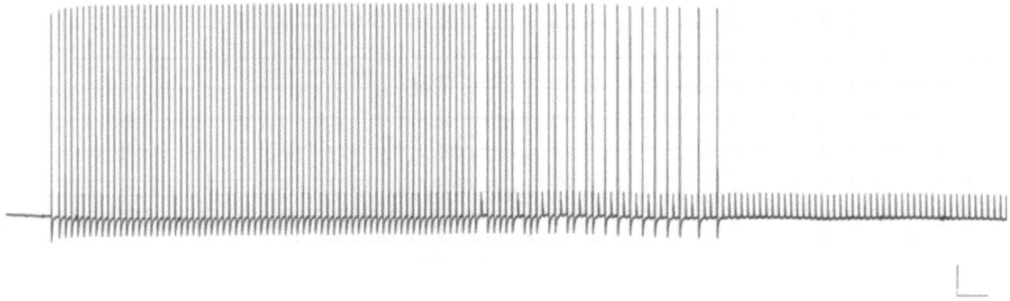

Fig. 2. Neuronal response to stimulation with intracellular current impulses. The neuron responded to stimulation with 93 AP after which all of the stimuli ceased to evoke an AP, Complete habituation was established and small depolarizing artefacts were present in recordings instead of the AP. The amplitude of the stimulus pulses was 0.7 nA. the width of the intracellular stimulating impulses was 4 msec. Current stimulating impulses are not shown because each of these impulses causes the firing of one AP or the appearance of one artefact on the recordings. The calibration is 10 mV, 5 s.

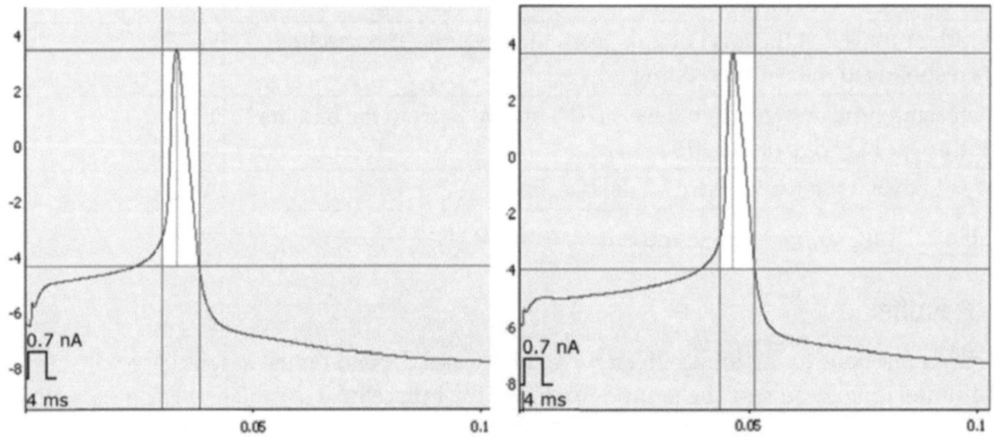

Fig. 3. The different AP parameters correspond to a different stimulus number:
a) AP fired by the neuron in response to the 1st intracellular current impulse. The parameters are: Latent period = 20.8 ms; W20 = 25.6 ms; Tr = 1.92 ms; Area = 0.106 V.s.
b) AP fired by the neuron in response to the 10th intracellular current impulse. The parameters are: Latent period = 33.6 ms; W20 = 33.6 ms; Tr = 2.56 ms; Area = 0.135 V.s. The broadening of the AP is evident. The intracellular stimulating impulses are schematically shown at the left lower corner of the recordings.

The parameters of the AP and the latent period varied irregularly during an increase of the number of the applied intracellular current impulses. The numerical values of AP parameters and the latent period trended to increase during an increase of the number of stimulating impulses (i.e. with an increase of the AP number, since the stimulus number coincides with the AP number). The typical dependence of the latent period, W20, Tr and Area on the stimulating impulse number (consequently on AP number) for one of the neurons is shown, respectively, in the Figures 4-7.

We determined the amount of information about habituation contained in the AP parameters (W20, Tr, Area) and the latent period. For this purpose, a mathematical model was selected for each parameter of the AP and the latent period. It was shown that this amount of information changes during an increase of the AP number. We deal with experimentally measured data. Consequently, it is essential that corresponding mathematical models have a stochastic character. In particular, sequences of latent periods and AP parameters (W20, Tr, Area) create a time series with a linear trend. According to the statistical investigations (the appendix), a time series with a linear trend represents a sufficiently good mathematical model. Concerning the time necessary for establishing habituation - it was not constant and it varied from neuron to neuron. Consequently, we obtained a numerical sequence containing 32 observed values of the time of habituation. The time of habituation might be regarded as a random variable. The theoretical mean value (mathematical expectation) of this random variable is unknown. A 99% confidence interval of this unknown mean value is 22, 45 -- 57, 49. The amount of information was experimentally calculated. The dynamics of the calculated information for the latent period are given in Figure 8. The information amount reaches its maximum value and then begins

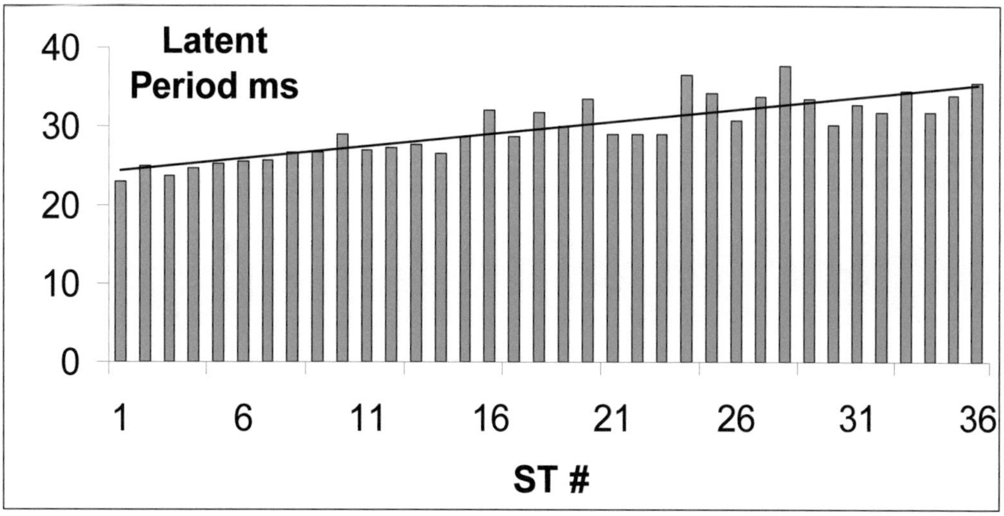

Fig. 4. An example of the latent period dependence on the stimulating impulse number for one neuron. On the abscissa, the number of intracellular stimulating impulses is plotted, while on the ordinate the latent period in milliseconds is plotted. Mean values of the measured latent period vary irregularly; however, the trend increases steadily. The amplitude of the applied intracellular current impulses was 0.1 nA and the duration of each of these impulse was 4 ms.

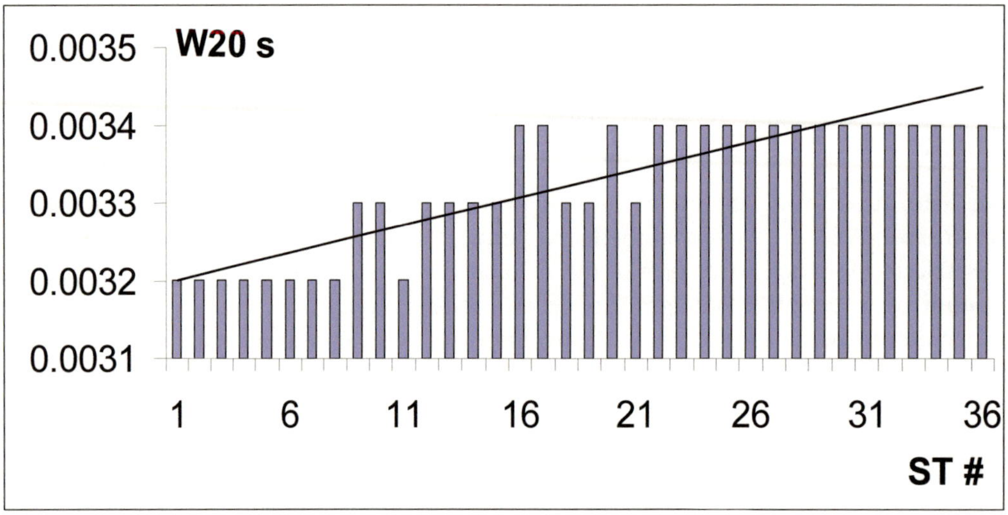

Fig. 5. An example of W20 dependence on the stimulating impulse number. On the abscissa is plotted the number of intracellular stimulating impulses, while on the ordinate is plotted W20 in seconds. The increase of the W20 is evident. The character of the trend is towards an increase. The amplitude of the applied intracellular current impulses was 0.1 nA, while the duration of each of these impulses was 4 ms.

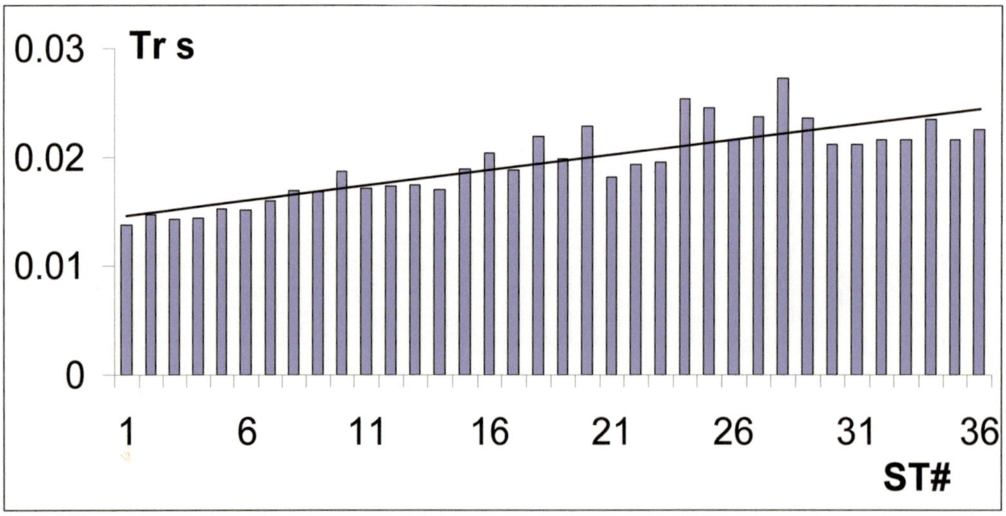

Fig. 6. Tr dependence on the stimulating impulse number. On the abscissa is plotted the number of intracellular stimulating impulses, while on the ordinate is plotted Tr in seconds. Tr varies irregularly, like the latent period. The trend also increases. The amplitude of the applied intracellular current impulses was 0.1 nA and the duration of each these was 4 ms.

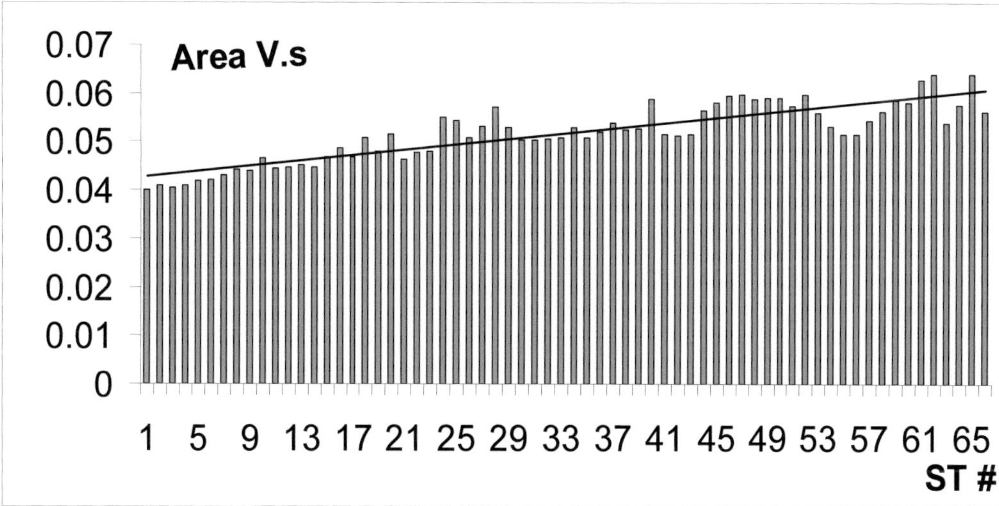

Fig. 7. Area dependence on the stimulating impulse number. On the abscissa is plotted the number of intracellular stimulating impulses, while on the ordinate is plotted the Area in Volt•seconds. The variations and trends are similar to the other parameters. The amplitude of the applied intracellular current impulses was 0.1 nA, while the duration of each of these pulses was 4 ms.

to decrease during the above mentioned 99% confidence interval. The dynamics of the calculated information for the other AP parameters were similar and, for this reason, are not shown here.

For more detailed consideration, let us consider the case of the latent period and then generalize it for the AP parameters. As is known (Yaglom & Yaglom, 1983), one random experiment contains some information about another random experiment. It is obvious that experiments must be interconnected. In our case, the first random experiment is the latent period's variation relative to its own trend. Let us denote this random experiment as experiment α. The second random experiment shows whether habituation is established. Let us denote this experiment as β.

The stimulating impulse numbers are plotted on the X axis. The amount of information contained in the α experiment in respect of the β experiment (i.e., about habituation) is plotted on the Y axis (Figure 8).

The number of the AP (which coincides with the stimulating impulse number) is plotted on the X axis. The calculated amount of information is plotted on the Y axis. As is noticeable, the amount of information firstly increases very quickly with an increase of the AP number. Then, the amount of information reaches a maximum value, after which it decreases. The 99% confidence interval is 22, 45 -- 57, 49. This confidence interval is shown through the lighter colouration.

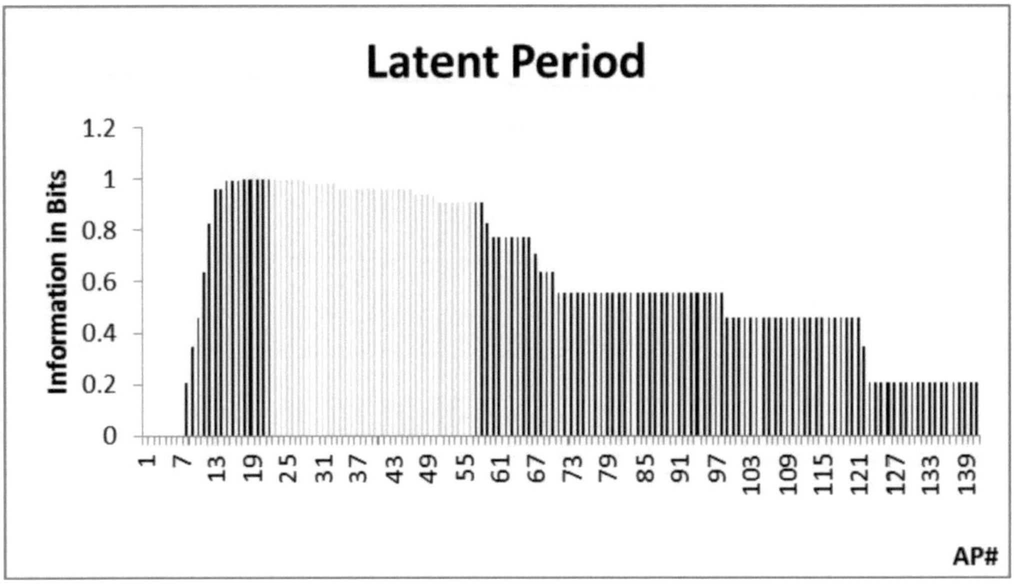

Fig. 8. Dependence of the amount of information on the AP number.

4. Discussion

Habituation is regarded as one form of learning (Kandel, 1976). Consequently, habituation might be understood as a result of the processing and saving of information. This phenomenon appears at different levels of the organism. Habituation also appears at the level of the individual neuron. Therefore, it could be stated that the observed effect of neuronal habituation in response to intracellular stimulation with current impulses might be thought of as a result of information processing at the level of the individual neuron.

We measured the defined quantities in our experiments. These quantities represent interconnected random variables. The variation of one of them inevitably causes the variation of the corresponding probability of the other random variable. Consequently, it is possible to speak about the amount of information which is contained in one random variable (random experiment) about another random variable.

As the parameters of the AP and the latent period are interconnected random variables, it is possible to calculate, experimentally, the amount of information with respect to the habituation contained in these variables.

The calculations show that an amount of information contained in each of the separate AP parameters or in the latent period differs from zero. Their behaviour is given by Figure 8. This enables one to discuss and analyse the semantics of the information; however, this is an issue for a separate study. In the present study, we are concerned only with changes of the amount of information and so we emphasise that the AP parameters contain certain information about habituation (habituation time).

Results similar to each other were observed for all variables. Particularly, at the beginning of stimulation up to the 7th - 10th application of intracellular current pulses the amount of information contained in the AP parameters or in the latent period is equal to zero- see figure 8. This means that 7-10 stimuli are not "understood" by the neuron as a signal that has to be learnt, i.e., to be habituated. With continuing stimulation, the amount of information begins to rapidly increase and reaches a value of approximately 1 bit. Although the absolutely value 1 bit is not high, nevertheless it shows that AP parameters and latent period are sensitive to information processing. Then the information begins to decline. This is also essential- apparently signals become "common" to the neuron and the amount of information begins to decrease. It might be speculated that a neuron does not receive more "new" information and "makes decision" to stop AP firing as a response to the stimulation (see the appendix).

As was mentioned above, the experiments revealed that the AP parameters and the latent period vary irregularly. Variation of any of these variables in time is well-described by the time series with a linear trend:

$$Y(t) = a + bt + \varepsilon(t),$$

where a and b are constant parameters, $t-$ is a time variable (the number of applied stimuli), $\varepsilon(t)$ is a random component with zero mathematical expectation. $Y(t)$ may be the latent period, W20, Tr, or Area. As the corresponding statistical procedures of hypothesis-testing confirm, all of the above mentioned variables display an increasing trend (see appendix).

It can be stated that the mechanisms producing the W20, Tr, Area and latent period are responsible for the process of information processing. The speculative explanation of the variation of the AP parameters and the latent period can be described as follows: the recurrent application of current stimulating impulses might increase the resistance of the membrane around the tip of the stimulus microelectrode. This, in turn, might reduce the amplitude of the perturbation of the membrane potential and slow down the electro-tonic propagation of the depolarization to the AP triggering zone. The result is an increase of the latent period and a broadening of the AP parameters. This, in turn, leads to habituation to intracellular stimulation.

5. Conclusion

A neuron habituates to repeated stimulation with intracellular current impulses. The parameters of an AP and the latency period vary during habituation (i.e., the waveform of the AP changes). These variations contain information about habituation. Therefore, the question "Is it possible that the AP waveform contains some information about habituation when a single neuron is stimulated intracellularly?" has to be answered positively.

6. Appendix

One and the same type of mathematical model is used for all of the variables - W20, Tr, Area and the latent period. The model is called a "time series with linear trend". Consequently, for the purpose of notational simplification, let us first consider the mathematical model of latent period variation and then generalize it for the AP parameters.

$$Y(t) = a + bt + \varepsilon(t), \tag{1}$$

Here: $Y(t)$ is the latent period, $t-$ is the number of intracellular impulses (its time variable), a and b are constant parameters and $\varepsilon(t)$ represents a random component with zero mathematical expectation. Experiments were performed on 32 neurons. Consequently, the latent period was measured in a series of 32 experiments. From formula (1), it is derived that the result of measurements for an ith series (i.e., for i[th] neuron) could be written as follows:

$$Y_i(t) = a_i^* + b_i^* t + \varepsilon_i(t),\, i = 1,2,...,32$$

where a_i^* and b_i^* represent statistical estimations of unknown a and b coefficients.

As is well known (Cramer, 1945), a_i^* and b_i^* are given by the following formulae:

$$b_i^* = \frac{\sum_{t=1}^{m_i} tY_i(t) - m_i\left(\frac{1+m_i}{2}\right)\overline{Y_i}}{\sum_{t=1}^{m_i} t^2 - m_i\left(\frac{1+m_i}{2}\right)^2}, \tag{2}$$

$$a_i^* = \overline{Y_i} - \frac{1+m_i}{2} b_i^*, \tag{3}$$

$$\overline{Y_i} = \frac{1}{m_i}\sum_{t=1}^{m_i} Y_i(t). \tag{4}$$

where m_i is the time of habituation for the ith neuron.

The adequacy of the selected model (1) must first be tested with statistical methods.

Let us introduce the notation $X(t) = a + bt$ for the linear trend. Consequently, we will have notations for observed data of the ith neuron, such that:

$$X_i^*(t) = a_i^* + b_i^* t, \quad i = 1,2,...,32$$

Let us consider the difference $\varepsilon(t) = Y(t) - X(t)$ for the testing of the adequacy of the model (1) and let us set the following task for hypothesis testing:

$H_0: \ E\varepsilon(t) = 0$ (main hypothesis),

$H_1: \ E\varepsilon(t) \neq 0$ (alternative hypothesis).

Here, $E\varepsilon(t)$ is the mathematical expectation for the fixed t.

Let us consider the differences $\varepsilon_i^*(t) = Y_i(t) - X_i^*(t), \ t = 1,2,...,m_i$ and the arithmetical mean comprised by these differences $\overline{\varepsilon_i^*} = \frac{1}{m_i}\sum_{t=1}^{m_i} \varepsilon_i^*(t)$ for each ith neuron for the purpose of conducting the hypothesis testing procedures (the so-called t test). Statistics $\overline{\varepsilon_1^*}, \overline{\varepsilon_2^*}, ..., \overline{\varepsilon_{32}^*}$ will then be obtained. Let us take the statistics $T = \frac{\overline{\varepsilon^*}}{s}\sqrt{32}$ as criteria statistics - so-called t statistics.

Here, $\overline{\varepsilon^*} = \frac{1}{32}\sum_{i=1}^{32} \overline{\varepsilon_i^*}$ and $s = \left(\frac{1}{31}\sum_{i=1}^{32}\left(\overline{\varepsilon_i^*}\right)^2 - \frac{32}{31}\left(\overline{\varepsilon^*}\right)^2 \right)^{1/2}$.

We use standard normal distribution tables because the statistical sample consists of the 32 terms and the corresponding tables of the t-statistics is comprised by not more than 30 terms from the sample. The corresponding calculation for the latent periods shows that the numerical value of the $t-$ statistics is approximately equal to -0.199, and the P value is approximately equal to 0.846. The above mentioned mathematical model was applied to the AP parameters also. The corresponding calculations show that:

1. Numerical value of t - statistics is -0.474 and P value is 0.64 for W20.
2. Numerical value of t - statistics is -0.531 and P value is 0.6 for Tr.
3. Numerical value of t - statistics is -0.232 and P value is 0.82 for Area.

It is obvious that the P values are sufficiently large in all cases. Consequently, it could be stated that there is no basis for discarding H_0 hypothesizes. This means, in turn, that the application of the mathematical model (1) of the time sequence is relevant for all AP parameters and the latent period. Now, let us consider the statistical hypothesis test for proving that there are increasing trends for the latent period and the AP parameters before establishing habituation. To avoid overloading the corresponding formulas with too much notation, let us provide a procedure of statistical hypothesis testing for the latent period (the so-called $t-$test). Then, generalize this t test for all of the AP parameters. Let us calculate statistical estimations b_i^* of the unknown b coefficients included in formula (1) by means of formula (2) for each ith neuron.

Statistics $b_1^*, b_2^*, ..., b_{32}^*$ will be obtained as a result. The statistical hypotheses

$H_0: b = 0$ (main hypothesis)

$H_1 : b > 0$ (alternative hypothesis)

must be tested based on these statistics. The alternative hypothesis obviously implies that the line of the trend is rising.

The numerical value of the so-called t statistics $T = \frac{\overline{b^*}}{s}\sqrt{32}$ has to be calculated for the use of the $t-$ test. Here, $\overline{b^*} = \frac{1}{32}\sum_{i=1}^{32} b_i^*$ and $s = \left(\frac{1}{31}\sum_{i=1}^{32}\left(b_i^*\right)^2 - \frac{32}{31}\left(\overline{b^*}\right)^2\right)^{1/2}$. The calculations show that the numerical value of the $t-$ statistics for the latent period is approximately equal to 2.77. The P value is approximately equal to 0.003.

For the AP parameters, similar calculations show that:

1. The numerical value of the t -statistics is 3.254. The P value is approximately equal to 0.0001 for the W20
2. The numerical value of the t -statistics is 2.498. The P value is approximately equal to 0.007 for the Tr.
3. The numerical value of the t -statistics is 3.07. The P value is approximately equal to 0.002 for the Area.

It is obvious that the P values are such small numbers that H_0 hypothesis must be discarded for the AP parameters and the latent period. Correspondingly, H_1 must be accepted. Therefore, it could be stated that the AP parameters and latent periods have an increasing trend. Let us calculate the amount of information. We take "α experiment" for the determination of the variable's location relative to its own trend (above or under) and "β experiment" for the determination of the habituation. Under the term "α experiment" we imply the results of measurements of the variables. Under the term "variables", values of the latent period, W20, Tr and Area are implied. Under the term "β experiment", we imply the determination of whether habituation is established. $I(\alpha,\beta) = H(\beta) - H_\alpha(\beta)$ is the amount of information retained in the "α experiment" regarding the "β experiment" – (Yaglom & Yaglom, 1983). Here, $H(\beta)$ is the entropy of the "β experiment" and $H_\alpha(\beta)$ is the conditional entropy of the "β experiment" in relation to the "α experiment". It is known that $H(\beta) = -P(B_1)\log_2 P(B_1) - P(B_2)\log_2 P(B_2)$. Here, B_1 is the state of affairs where habituation exists, while B_2 is the state of affairs where habituation is absent.

Correspondingly:

$$H_\alpha(\beta) = P(A_1)H_{A_1}(\beta) + P(A_2)H_{A_2}(\beta)$$

$$H_{A_i}(\beta) = -P_{A_i}(B_1)\log_2 P_{A_i}(B_1) - P_{A_i}(B_2)\log_2 P_{A_i}(B_2),\ i = 1,2$$

Here A_1 is state of affairs where the numerical value is over the trend line, while A_2 is the state of affairs where the numerical value is under the trend line. In our experiments, the amount of information depends upon the stimulating impulse number n. For this reason, $I_n(\alpha,\beta)$ will be written instead of $I(\alpha,\beta)$. We are interested in the amount of information's behaviour during increase of n. The charts of the amount of information $I_n(\alpha,\beta)$ are obtained as a result of experimental calculations of the above given probabilities $P(A_i),P(B_i),P_{A_i}(B_j), i,j=1,2$. The stimulating impulse numbers are plotted on the abscissa axis, while the numerical values of the amount of information $I_n(\alpha,\beta)$ are plotted on the ordinate axis in these charts. As these charts show, the amount of information increases up to certain value, and then it decreases and habituation increases. It might be stated that after a certain number of stimulating impulses no "novelty" occurs for the neuron, and so the amount of information decreases and habituation increases.

7. References

Arakelov, G. Marakujieva, I. & Palikhova, T. (1991). Structural and functional analysis of monosynaptic connections between identified neurons of Helix lucorum. *Simpler nervous systems* (Eds. D.A. Sakharov and W. Winlow), pp. 258-269, University Press, Manchester.

Cramer, H. (1945). *Mathematical methods of statistics.* Almqvist & Wiksells, Uppsala.

De Polavieja, G. Harsch, A. Kleppe, I. Robinson, H. & Juusola, M. (2005). Stimulus History Reliably Shapes Waveforms of Cortical Neurons. *J. Neurosci.* Vol. 25, No. 23 , pp. 5657–5665.

Gerstner, W. & Kistler, W. (2002). *Spiking Neuron Models. Single Neurons, Populations, Plasticity, 2002.* Available from: http://icwww.epfl.ch/~gerstner/SPNM/node8.html

Häusser, M. Major, G. & Stuart, G. (2001). Differential shunting of EPSPs by Action Potentials. *Science* Vol. 291, No. 5501 pp. 138-141.

Juusola, M. Robinson, H. & de Polavieja, G. (2007). Coding with spike shapes and graded potentials in cortical networks. *Bioessays* Vol. 29, No. 2, pp. 178-187.

Kandel, E. (1976). *Cellular Basis of Behavior,* W.H. Freeman & Company, San Francisco.

Koch, C. (1999). *Biophysics of Computation,* Oxford Univ. Press, ISBN, New York.

Koch, C. & Segev, I. (2000). The role of single neurons in information processing, Nature Neurosience, Vol. 3, No. Supp, pp. 1171-1177.

Partsvania, B. Shoshiashvili, L. Sulaberidze T. & Modebadze, Z. (2008). Extremely Low Frequency Magnetic Fields effects on the Snail Single Neurons. *Electromagnetic biology and Medicine.* Vol. 27, No. 4, pp. 409-418.

Robinson, H. (1994). Conductance injection. *Trends Neurosci.* Vol. 17, No. 4, pp. 147-148.

Shu, Y. Hasenstaub, A. Duque A. Yu, Y. & McCormick, D. (2006). Modulation of intracortical synaptic potentials by presynaptic somatic membrane potential. *Nature.* Vol. 441, No. 7094, pp. 761-765.

Tateno, T. & Robinson, H. (2006). Rate Coding and Spike-Time Variability in Cortical Neurons with Two Types of Threshold Dynamics. *J. Neurophysiol.* Vol. 95, No. 4, pp. 2650-2663.

Yaglom, A. & Yaglom, I. (1983). *Probability and Information.* Reidel Publishing Co., Delhi.

2

Electrophysiological Recording and Imaging of Neuronal Signals in Brain Slices

Thomas Heinbockel
Department of Anatomy,
Howard University College of Medicine, Washington,
USA

1. Introduction

A pressing issue in our understanding of neuronal circuitry is the functional significance of neuromodulator systems. Recent experiments in brain slices that employed new methods and technical innovations have described novel aspects of classic brain signaling mechanisms or revealed unknown mechanisms of cellular communication involving specific neuromodulator systems. Here, we focus on two of these systems, (1) the neurotransmitter glutamate and its metabotropic receptors and (2) novel brain signaling molecules, endocannabinoids, and their receptors, cannabinoid receptors. The study of these two neuromodulator systems has been greatly aided by technological advances in recording and imaging techniques. We describe these techniques and present data to illustrate how these two neuromodulator systems regulate intrinsic properties of neurons and shape sensory and synaptic responses of neurons in the olfactory (main olfactory bulb, MOB) and limbic system (hippocampus).

The first part of this review will focus on electrophysiological recording and imaging techniques that helped to study the amino acid glutamate as the principal excitatory neurotransmitter in the MOB of the brain. The MOB is the first relay station in the CNS for processing sensory information that comes from olfactory receptor neurons in the nasal epithelium. Neuroanatomical studies demonstrate that projection neurons (mitral and tufted cells) as well as inhibitory interneurons such as GABAergic granule cells in the MOB express high levels of metabotropic glutamate receptors (mGluRs), suggesting that these receptors play a role in the function of the MOB network. Olfactory nerve terminals synapse onto MOB projection neurons, which is mediated by glutamate acting at AMPA and NMDA ionotropic glutamate receptor (iGluR) subtypes as well as mGluRs. New experiments in the MOB have used patch-clamp recordings, microsurgery, optical-imaging (voltage-sensitive dye imaging) and use of mGluR gene knockout mice. These experiments have illuminated the role of mGluRs in the MOB and point toward novel and potent regulatory roles of these receptors in shaping olfactory output from the MOB to higher olfactory centers in the brain.

The second part of this review will concentrate on electrophysiological recording and imaging techniques that have established the role of retrograde signaling by endocannabinoids in the hippocampus. Cannabinoids are the active ingredient of marijuana. In addition to being known and used as recreational drugs, cannabinoids are produced endogenously by neurons in the brain (endocannabinoids) and serve as important signaling molecules in the nervous system and the rest of the body. A combination of patch-clamp electrophysiology in cultured brain slices, calcium measurements, and flash photolysis of novel caged compounds has allowed determining the temporal kinetics of the hippocampal endocannabinoid signaling cascade.

2. Synaptic signaling in the Main Olfactory Bulb

The development of an acute slice preparation of the rodent MOB has greatly improved the functional exploration and understanding of the mammalian olfactory system (Shipley and Ennis, 1996). The intrinsic MOB circuitry is functionally preserved in MOB slice preparations (~400 µm thickness). The axon of each olfactory receptor neuron projects through the olfactory nerve layer (ONL) of the MOB and allows electrical stimulation of afferent inputs (Fig. 1). The functional layers of the MOB and their intrinsic cell types can easily be identified visually. Likewise, axons of output neurons, mitral/tufted cells, leaving the MOB through the lateral olfactory tract (LOT) can be accessed (Nickell et al, 1994; Liu et al, 1994; Aroniadou-Anderjaska et al, 1997; Keller et al, 1998; Aroniadou-Anderjaska et al, 1999). Microdissection cuts in MOB slices allow to isolate specific synaptic pathways, generate slices that contain only selected layers of the MOB (Aungst et al, 2003) or preserve axon pathways projecting back into the MOB from olfactory cortex (Laaris et al, 2007; Balu et al, 2007). These preparations have permitted studying specific synaptic pathways at different levels of processing using electrophysiological and imaging techniques. In the

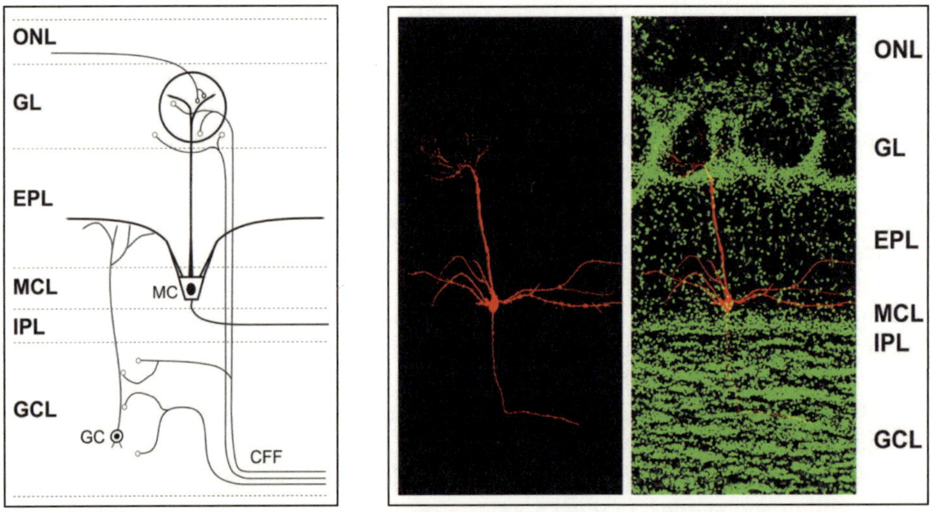

Fig. 1. Left panel: Simplified diagram of the MOB to illustrate neuronal elements under study (mitral and granule cells). For clarity, other cell types have been omitted from the diagram. EPL - external plexiform layer, GCL - granule cell layer, GL - glomerular layer, IPL - internal plexiform layer, ONL - olfactory nerve layer, MCL - mitral cell layer, MC - mitral cell, GC - granule cell, CFF - centrifugal fibers. Right: Confocal micrograph of a section of the adult mouse main olfactory bulb with a single mitral cell intracellularly filled with biocytin (red) and nuclei stained with counterstain Sytox Green (green). The mitral cell soma is located in the mitral cell layer (MCL). One apical dendrite reaches into one glomerulus and several lateral dendrites span the MOB. Mitral cells are key output neurons from the MOB. Modified from Heinbockel and Ennis, 2008.

MOB, glutamate is the major excitatory neurotransmitter. Synapses in the MOB most often are formed as serial or reciprocal glutamatergic/GABAergic circuits in discrete layers of the tissue, typically between dendrites of MOB output neurons and local interneurons (reviewed in Heinbockel and Heyward, 2009).

2.1 Metabotropic glutamate receptors in the Main Olfactory Bulb

Metabotropic glutamate receptors are expressed at unusually high density in the MOB (reviewed in Ennis et al, 2007). Selective mGluR pharmacological reagents as well as mGluR-specific knockout mice have revealed a wide variety of physiological responses and ion channels that are modulated by mGluRs (Conn and Pin, 1997; Schoepp et al, 1999). Eight mGluR subtypes have been cloned and are subdivided into three groups based on second messenger linkage, sequence homology and pharmacological sensitivity of the receptors: Group I (mGluR1 & mGluR5), Group II (mGluR2 & mGluR3) and Group III (mGluR4, mGluR6, mGluR7 & mGluR8). Six of these eight mGluR subtypes have been found in the MOB (reviewed in Heinbockel and Ennis, 2008). While many functions of ionotropic glutamate receptors in the MOB are now well understood (reviewed in Heinbockel and Heyward, 2009), relatively little is known about the function of mGluRs. Recent experiments that employed a combination of patch-clamp electrophysiology, voltage-sensitive dye imaging, and use of mGluR gene knockout mice have determined the role of mGluRs in the MOB and demonstrate potent regulatory roles of these receptors in shaping MOB synaptic output (Heinbockel and Ennis, 2008; Dong et al., 2009).

mGluRs and iGluRs are distinctly different in their mode of ion channel regulation and time course of action as well as in their sensitivity to glutamate (ED_{50}: mGluR1, 5: 10 µM; AMPAR: 200-500 µM; NMDAR: 2.5-3 µM) (Meldrum, 2000). mGluRs can be much more sensitive to glutamate than iGluRs (AMPA receptors), even though the ED_{50} for glutamate at AMPA/kainate receptors is significantly determined by subunit composition (Dingledine et al, 1999; Meldrum, 2000). This has important functional consequences for tonic mGluR activation and sensitivity to glutamate spillover under conditions where glutamate concentrations are too low to activate AMPA receptors.

Mitral and tufted cells express high levels of mGluR1 (Masu et al, 1991; Martin et al, 1992; Shigemoto et al, 1992; van den Pol, 1995; Sahara et al, 2001) (Figs. 1, 3). mGluR1 is present on the cell body, and apical and lateral dendrites of mitral and tufted cells, and the splice variant mGluR1a has been localized postsynaptically at olfactory nerve synapses (van den Pol, 1995) which suggests that mGluR1 mediates responses of mitral and tufted cells to glutamatergic inputs from olfactory nerve terminals, and/or could function as auto- or heteroreceptors for glutamate released from the apical or lateral dendrites of mitral and tufted cells. In contrast to their counterparts in the accessory olfactory bulb (where responses to pheromones are processed in many mammals), mitral and tufted cells in the MOB do not express Group II receptors (mGluR2/3) (Ohishi et al, 1993; 1998). mGluR7 and mGluR8 are present on the axon terminals of mitral and tufted cells in piriform cortex (Kinzie et al, 1995; Saugstad et al, 1997; Kinoshita et al, 1998; Wada et al, 1998).

Granule cells express mGluR5 (Group I) (Romano et al., 1995). mGluR5 staining is strongest in the granule cell layer where cell bodies of granule cells are located (Sahara et al., 2001). mGluR5 is found on portions of granule cell dendrites in the external plexiform layer (EPL) apposed to presynaptic glutamatergic synapses from mitral and tufted cell lateral dendrites (van den Pol, 1995). mGluR5 may mediate, at least in part, responses of granule cells to glutamatergic inputs from mitral and tufted cells. Granule cells in the granule cell layer do not express mGluR1 (van den Pol, 1995; Heinbockel et al., 2004). Immunocytochemistry shows only weak staining for mGluR1 (Martin et al. 1992; Sahara et al. 2001; van den Pol 1995), and in situ hybridization reveals faint mGluR1 expression (Shigemoto et al. 1992). Instead, granule cells may express low to moderate levels of mGluR2 (Group II, Ohishi et al., 1993, 1998), and low levels of mGluR4 and mGluR7 (Group III; Kinzie et al., 1995; Ohishi et al., 1995; Saugstad, 1997; Wada et al., 1998).

Given the abundant expression in MOB neurons and in light of the limited knowledge of mGluR function, a pressing issue in the organization and operation of the olfactory system is the analysis of mGluR actions on adult MOB neurons and upon MOB network function. For several reasons, the MOB is an ideal platform for investigating how mGluRs modulate neural network dynamics to enhance sensory processing. (1) Output neurons in the MOB receive direct sensory input, even though this input is strongly modified by intrinsic inhibitory interneurons that provide two discrete tiers for lateral interactions, namely, in the glomerular layer and in the external plexiform layer. (2) Vast cortical and subcortical centrifugal inputs project to the MOB and modulate local circuit processing at multiple levels. (3) The structural organization and the diverse neuronal input-output relationships make the MOB preparation distinctly different from hippocampus, amygdala, neocortex, and cerebellum for addressing functional questions of mGluR modulation in the brain. mGluRs in these and other brain regions are involved in diseases such as stroke, epilepsy, Alzheimer's, Parkinson's and Huntington's disease, as well as in pain, schizophrenia, and anxiety (Lea and Faden, 2003; Schoepp and Conn, 1993). Consequently, our studies about the mechanisms through which mGluR activation shapes synaptic information in a model neural circuit such as the MOB helps to fill major gaps in our understanding of the functioning of both the olfactory system and other brain regions.

2.2 Main Olfactory Bulb slice preparation, recording and imaging techniques

In order to prepare acute slices of the MOB, we used commercially available male and female rats (Sprague-Dawley; Zivic Laboratories, Zelienople, PA) and mice (C57Bl/6J, Jackson Laboratory, Bar Harbor, ME) and mGluR1 and mGluR5 mutant mice (C57Bl/6J background) (Chiamulera et al. 2001; Conquet et al. 1994) from our colony. mGluR5 mice were provided as a homozygous mutant line, whereas mGluR1 mice, generated as a lacZ knock-in, were maintained by heterozygous mating and were genotyped by polymerase chain reaction (PCR) of DNA from tail tip digests (Heinbockel et al., 2004). Homozygous mGluR1 mutant mice were also identified phenotypically by their characteristic progressive mobility deficit at several weeks of age (Conquet et al. 1994).

We used conventional immunohistochemical techniques to map the distribution of neurons expressing β-galactosidase (β-gal) in tissue sections harvested from mGluR1 transgenic animals (Heinbockel et al., 2004). Sections were examined under brightfield optics using a Leica DMRX photomicroscope (Leica, Deerfield, IL). Digital microscopy images were captured using a Phase I digital camera (PhaseOne, Northport, NY), sized, and balanced for brightness and contrast using Adobe Photoshop 5.0 (Adobe Systems, San Jose, CA).

Juvenile (21- to 31-day old) rats or mice were decapitated, the MOBs dissected out and immersed in artificial cerebrospinal fluid (ACSF) at 4°C (Heinbockel et al., 2004, 2007a, b).

Horizontal slices (400-μm-thick) of the MOB were cut parallel to its long axis using a vibratome (Vibratome Series 1000, Ted Pella, Redding, CA). After a period of recovery (30 min) at 30°C, the slices were incubated in a holding bath at room temperature (22°C) until used. For recording, a single brain slice was placed in a perfusion-bath recording chamber mounted on a microscope stage and maintained at 30 ± 0.5°C. Slices were submerged in ACSF flowing at 2.5-3 ml/min.

Visually guided recordings from neurons in the mitral cell layer or granule cell layer were made with near-infrared differential interference contrast (NIR DIC) optics, water-immersion objectives, and a BX50WI microscope (Olympus Optical, Tokyo) (Stuart et al. 1993). NIR transillumination was at 900 nm (filter transmission, 850–950 nm) concentric with the objective and optimized for DIC. A 0.25-in CCD camera (CCD 100, Dage, Stamford, CT), fitted with a 3-to-1 zooming coupler (Optem, Fairport, NY) was used. Contrast was enhanced in real-time using an image processor (Model 794, Hughes Aircraft Company, Carlsbad, CA) and the image was displayed on a monochrome monitor (Dage HR120, Dage-MTI, Michigan City, IN).

Recordings were made using conventional whole cell patch-clamp methods. Recording pipettes were pulled on a Flaming-Brown P-97 puller (Sutter Instrument, Novato, CA) from standard-wall filamented 1.5-mm-diameter borosilicate glass; tip diameter was 2–3 μm, tip resistance was 5–8 MΩ. Seal resistance was routinely >1GΩ and liquid junction potential was 9-10 mV; reported measurements were not corrected for this potential. Data were obtained using a Multiclamp 700B amplifier (Molecular Devices, Sunnyvale, CA). Signals were low-pass Bessel filtered at 2 kHz and digitized on computer disc (Clampex 10.1, Molecular Devices). Data were also collected through a Digidata 1440A Interface (Molecular Devices) and digitized at 10 kHz. Holding currents were generated under control of the Multiclamp 700B Commander. Membrane resistance was calculated from the amount of steady-state current required to hyperpolarize the cell by 10 mV, typically from -60 mV to -70 mV.

To allow histological confirmation of recorded cells, biocytin (0.05% to 0.1%, Molecular Probes) was added to the pipette solution in some experiments. The presence of biocytin had no evident effect on neuronal electrophysiology. After recording, slices were fixed overnight in phosphate-buffered 4% paraformaldehyde at 4°C. Slices were incubated with Cy3-conjugated Streptavidin (Jackson ImmunoResearch Laboratories) and processed for later visualization and cell identification with laser-scanning confocal microscopy (FluoView confocal microscope, Olympus Instruments, Long Beach, CA) as described previously (Puche and Shipley 2001).

Since the axon of each olfactory receptor neuron projected through the olfactory nerve layer, it was possible in the MOB slice preparation to mimic olfactory stimulation by electrically stimulating afferent inputs. The olfactory nerve layer was focally stimulated with a bipolar electrode constructed from a pair of twisted stainless-steel wires (70 μm), insulated except for bluntly cut tips. The tips of the wires were placed tangentially along the peripheral surface of the olfactory nerve layer, slightly rostral to the estimated location of the recorded MC. Stimuli were isolated monophasic square wave pulses (10–200 μA in amplitude, 0.1 ms in duration) delivered by a Grass S8800 stimulator (Astro-Med, West Warwick, RI) and an isolated constant current source (Grass PSIU6, Astro-Med).

The ACSF used for perfusion of slices in the recording bath consisted of (in mM) 120 NaCl, 3 KCl, 1.3 $CaCl_2$, 1.3 $MgSO_4$, 10 glucose, 25 $NaHCO_3$, and 5 *N,N*-bis(2-hydroxyethyl)-2-

aminoethanesulfonic acid (BES), 95% O_2-5% CO_2-saturated, pH 7.27, 300 mOsm (Heinbockel et al., 2004). Recording pipettes were filled with the following solution (in mM) 125 K gluconate, 2 $MgCl_2$, 10 HEPES, 2 Mg_2ATP, 0.2 Na_3GTP, 1 NaCl, and 0.2 EGTA.

Optical imaging of voltage-sensitive dye signals was used to investigate network activity patterns evoked by stimulation of the lateral olfactory tract (LOT) (Heinbockel et al., 2007a). Slices were harvested as described above for electrophysiological recording. Slices were kept at room temperature in ACSF and stained with the voltage-sensitive dye RH-414 (100 µM; Molecular Probes, Eugene, OR) dissolved in ACSF. A single slice was placed in a static bath containing the dye solution, continuously aerated with 95% O_2-5% CO_2 for 30–45 min. Subsequently, the stained slice was transferred to an immersion-type recording chamber and continuously perfused at 2 ml/min with ACSF at room temperature. Unbound dye was washed out from stained slices by perfusion with ACSF for ≥15 min prior to optical recording. Methods used for recording voltage-sensitive optical signals were similar to those described in detail by Keller et al., 1998 and Laaris et al., 2007. Light from a 100 W tungsten-halogen lamp was band-limited with interference (540 ± 30 nm band-pass, Omega Optical, Brattleboro, VT) and heat filters. A 10x water-immersion objective (Olympus) was used to collect light from the preparation and projected onto a hexagonal 464 element array of photodiodes (NeuroPlex, OptImaging, Fairfield, CT). An individual photodiode sampled optical signals from a region of ~60 x 60 μm^2. Current output from each photodiode was separately converted to voltages, amplified in two separate stages (x1,000), multiplexed, and digitized at 12-bit resolution with an A/D converter. Before digitizing, optical signals were filtered at 500 Hz. Collection of optical signals was at a sampling rate of 1.63 kHz. Data were recorded and saved on a personal computer controlled by NeuroPlex software (OptImaging). Data analysis was performed on an Apple Macintosh computer, using routines developed in Igor (WaveMetrics, Lake Oswego, OR). A custom-designed beam splitting device (Microscope Services, Rockville, MD) was used to simultaneously project the images of the slice and light from light-emitting diodes embedded in the photodiode array onto the image plane of a CCD camera (Dage CCD72, Michigan City, IN). This allowed for the precise identification of the regions in the slice from which optical recordings were collected. Thus, this setup helped to correlate voltage-sensitive dye optical signals with the laminar borders of different layers in MOB slices (Figs. 1, 7).

2.3 Activation of mitral cells in the Main Olfactory Bulb by a selective group I mGluR agonist

Since little was known about the physiological role of Group I mGluRs on mitral cells, the first step was to determine the actions of Group I mGluRs on mitral cell excitability and responsiveness to sensory input from olfactory receptor neuron terminals. To experimentally approach these issues, we studied the consequences of activation or blockade of mGluRs on mitral cells. The data demonstrated an important role of mGluR1 in regulating the excitability of mitral cells (Heinbockel et al., 2004). A selective Group I mGluR agonist ((RS)-3,5-dihydroxyphenylglycine [DHPG]) potently and dose dependently depolarized (14 mV) and increased the firing rate of mitral cells (Fig. 2). Neither a Group II agonist (2S,3S,4S)-CCG/(2S,1'S,2'S)-2-(carboxycyclopropyl)glycine (L-CCG-I) nor a Group III agonist L(+)-2-amino-4-phosphonobutyric acid (AP4) depolarized mitral cells or increased their firing rates. The Group II and III agonist, L-CCG-I and AP4, did not evoke significant shifts of the holding current in voltage clamp recordings. The effects of DHPG

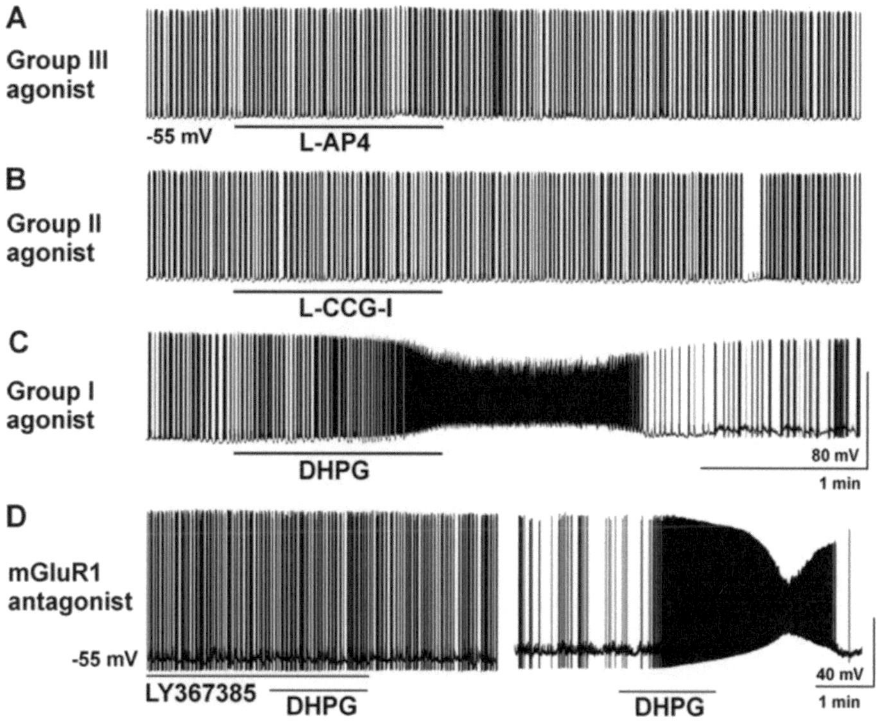

Fig. 2. Bath application of the Group I mGluR agonist DHPG activated mitral cells whereas the selective mGluR1 antagonist LY367385 blocked the effect of DHPG (C, D). A, B: Group II and III mGluR agonists had no effect on firing and membrane potential of mitral cells. Modified from Heinbockel et al., 2004 with permission of The American Physiological Society.

were a result of direct activation of mGluR1 on mitral cells as they persisted in the presence of blockers of synaptic transmission (NMDA receptor blocker [DL-2-amino-5-phosphonopentanoic acid (APV)], AMPA receptor blocker [6-cyano-7-nitroquinoxaline-2-3-dione (CNQX)], and $GABA_A$ receptor blocker [gabazine]) and/or TTX. The effects of DHPG were blocked by a preferential mGluR1 antagonist, LY367385, which has negligible actions on Group II and III mGluRs, and antagonizes mGluR5 only at concentrations in excess of 100 µM (Clark et al., 1997; Salt et al., 1999).

2.4 mGluR-mediated excitation of mitral cells in mGluR5 knockout mice and not in mGluR1 knockout mice

The specificity of mGluR agonists and antagonists is limited and can vary with concentration. Therefore, we took advantage of mice with targeted deletion of the mGluR1 receptor gene to further investigate the function of this receptor subtype on mitral cells (Conquet et al. 1994). In this transgenic strain, the mGluR1 gene sequence has been replaced with that for β-galactosidase (β-gal) by homologous recombination. Therefore, in "knockout" (KO) mice β-gal is present only in cells that would normally express mGluR1. We first examined the location of β-gal-positive (β-gal+) neurons in mGluR1 KO and wild-type (WT) littermate mice using immunohistochemistry. As shown in Fig. 3, the distribution of β-gal+

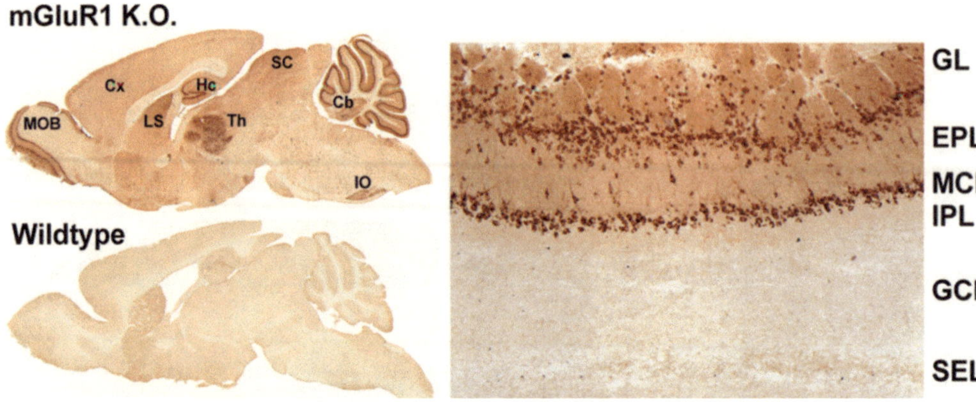

Fig. 3. mGluR1 distribution in KO and WT mice. Conventional immunohistochemical techniques were used to map the distribution of neurons expressing β-galactosidase (β-gal) in tissue sections harvested from mGluR1 transgenic animals. In this transgenic strain, the mGluR1 gene sequence had been replaced with that for β-galactosidase (β-gal) by homologous recombination; i.e., in KO mice β-gal is present only in cells that would normally express mGluR1. In sections of mGluR1 mutant (-/-) mice, β-gal staining was prominent in the cerebellum (Cb), hippocampus (Hc), thalamus (Th), lateral septum (LS), superior colliculus (SC), inferior olive (IO), main olfactory bulb (MOB), and throughout the cortex (Cx). In the MOB, strong and uniform staining was present in mitral cells. Tufted-like cells in the external plexiform layer, juxtaglomerular cells in the glomerular layer proper and at the glomerular layer-external plexiform layer border were also robustly stained. By contrast, no staining was observed in the internal plexiform or granule cell layers. β-gal staining was absent in mGluR1 WT littermates. GL - glomerular layer; EPL - external plexiform layer; MCL - mitral cell layer; IPL - internal plexiform layer; GCL - granule cell layer; SEL - subependymal layer. From Heinbockel et al., 2004; with permission of The American Physiological Society.

neurons in the MOB and other brain structures is consistent with previous reports on the distribution of mGluR1 (Martin et al. 1992; Petralia et al. 1997; Sahara et al. 2001; Shigemoto et al. 1992; van den Pol 1995). In the MOB (Fig. 3), strong and uniform staining is present in mitral cells. Tufted-like cells in the external plexiform layer and juxtaglomerular cells in the glomerular layer proper and at the glomerular layer-external plexiform layer border were also robustly stained. By contrast, no staining was observed in the internal plexiform or granule cell layers. β-gal staining was absent in mGluR1 WT littermates (Fig. 3). Excitatory actions of mGluR agonists on mitral cells were absent in mGluR1 knockout mice but were present in mGluR5 knockout mice (Fig. 4).

2.5 mGluR effects on intrinsic granule cell properties: Direct and indirect effects

Granule cells in the MOB are the largest population of GABAergic inhibitory interneurons. They modulate and shape the output of the MOB to higher-order olfactory structures (Shepherd et al., 2004). The apical dendrites of granule cells extend radially into the external plexiform layer, where they form dendrodendritic synapses with mitral and tufted cells (Fig. 1). Since granule cells express the highest level of mGluR5 in the brain (Romano et al., 1995), we hypothesized that mGluRs modulate granule cell excitability and responsiveness to glutamatergic synaptic input from mitral and tufted cells and, as a result, modulate granule

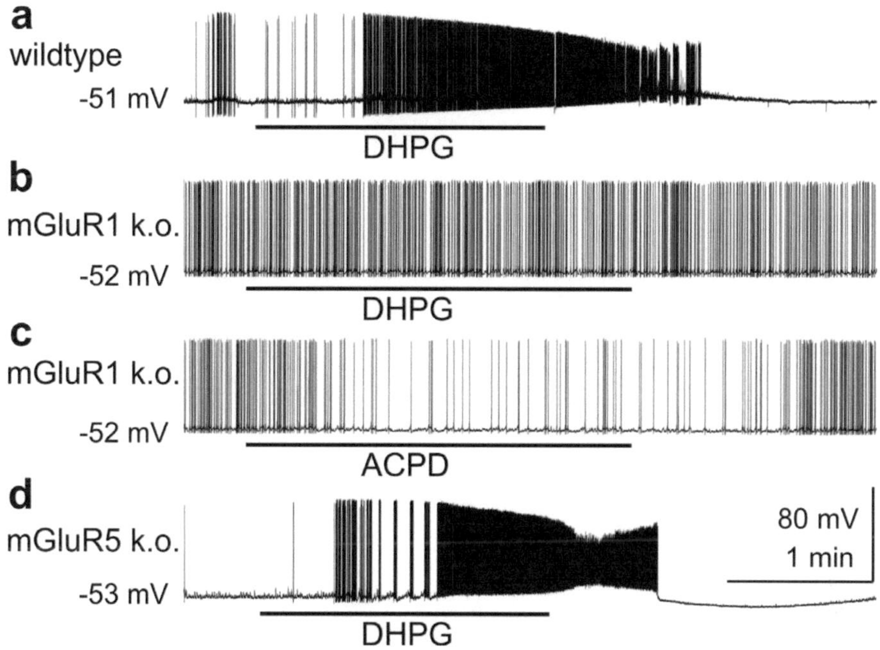

Fig. 4. Excitatory actions of mGluR agonists on mitral cells were absent in mGluR1 null mutant mice. a: Mitral cells recorded in slices harvested from wildtype mice are uniformly activated by the Group I mGluR agonist DHPG [(RS)-3,5-dihydroxyphenylglycine]. b: DHPG was without effect in mitral cells recorded in slices from mGluR1 null mutant (k.o.) mice. c: In contrast to its excitatory effect in wildtype mice, ACPD elicited a modest reduction in the firing rate of mitral cells recorded in slices from mGluR1 mutant (k.o.) mice. d: The excitatory effect of DHPG on mitral cells recorded in slices from mGluR5 null mutant (k.o.) mice was similar to that observed in wildtype mice. All experiments performed in the presence ionotropic (NMDA, AMPA) and $GABA_A$ receptor blockers, CNQX, APV, and gabazine, respectively. From Heinbockel et al., 2004; with permission of The American Physiological Society.

cell-mediated GABAergic inhibition of mitral and tufted cells. Therefore, we tested the consequences of activation or blockade of mGluR5 on granule cells using whole-cell patch clamp recordings and voltage-sensitive dye imaging in MOB slices from rats, wildtype mice, and mice with targeted gene deletions of Group I mGluRs.

Activation of mGluR5 directly increased the excitability of GABAergic granule cells located in the granule cell layer (deep granule cells) (Fig. 5), whereas inactivation of mGluR5 had opposite effects (Heinbockel et al., 2007a, b). The results indicated that mGluR5 modulated the strength of granule cell responses to glutamatergic inputs from mitral/tufted cells and granule cell-mediated dendrodendritic feedback inhibition in the MOB. Activation of mGluR5 by glutamate released from mitral/tufted cells could amplify lateral inhibition and, thereby, may increase contrast in the MOB network.

Without blockers of synaptic transmission, the Group I, II mGluR agonist ACPD or the Group I mGluR agonist DHPG depolarized (~20 mV) and increased the firing rate of granule cells (Fig. 5). These effects were direct and indirect in nature. mGluR5 on granule cells was directly activated by ACPD or DHPG. mGluR1 was activated on mitral cells and evoked an increase in glutamate release which in turn activated granule cells (indirect activation). In the presence of synaptic blockers, the mGluR agonists still depolarized granule cells, although the effect was reduced in amplitude. This result indicated that ACPD and DHPG directly depolarized granule cells.

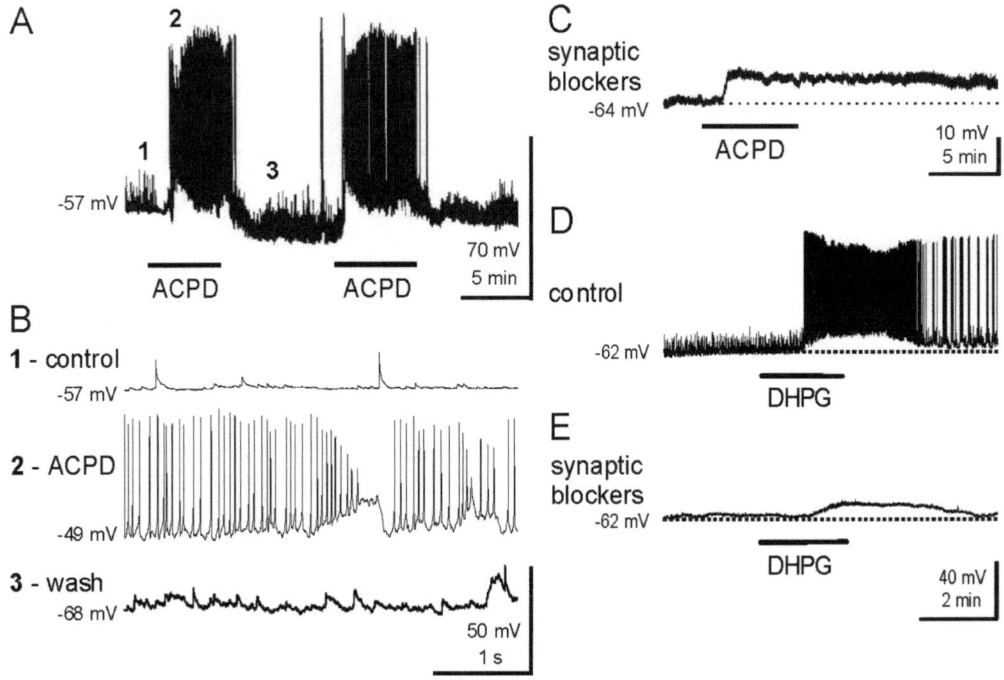

Fig. 5. mGluR agonists depolarized and increased the firing rate of granule cells. A, B: Response of a granule cell to the Group I, II mGluR agonist ACPD, shown at extended time scale in (B). Traces 1-3 correspond to timepoints in (A). C: In blockers of synaptic transmission the cell in (A) had reduced baseline spontaneous synaptic activity and a smaller response to ACPD. D, E: DHPG activated another granule cell. Blockers of synaptic transmission reduced baseline spontaneous synaptic activity (spontaneous EPSCs) and DHPG evoked a more moderate depolarization. From Heinbockel et al., 2007a; with permission of The American Physiological Society.

The direct actions of ACPD and DHPG on granule cells were mediated exclusively via activation of mGluR5 as shown by several lines of evidence. (1) The mGluR1 antagonist LY367385 did not block the effect of DHPG on granule cells, whereas it completely eliminated DHPG-evoked, mGluR1-mediated excitation of mitral cells at identical concentrations (Fig. 2) (Heinbockel et al., 2004). (2) DHPG had no discernible effects on granule cells in mGluR5 knockout mice, while it readily activated granule cells in mGluR1 knockout mice (Heinbockel et al., 2007b). (3) The Group II or Group III mGluR agonists evoked no currents in granule cells.

2.6 Activation of mGluR5 increases GABAergic inhibition of mitral cells

Excitatory mGluR5s on granule cells may facilitate feedback and feedforward inhibition of mitral cells. The question arose if mGluR5-evoked excitation of granule cells was sufficient to increase GABA release onto mitral cells? To address this question, we used voltage-clamp recordings to determine if DHPG-evoked activation of granule cells altered GABAergic inhibitory input to mitral cells. A high concentration of chloride was used in the patch pipette to increase the detectibility of IPSCs; under these conditions IPSCs appeared as inward currents. In the presence of iGluRblockers (i.e., blockers of AMPA and NMDA receptors), DHPG increased the frequency of IPSCs in mitral cells in wild-type mice (Fig. 6A). However,

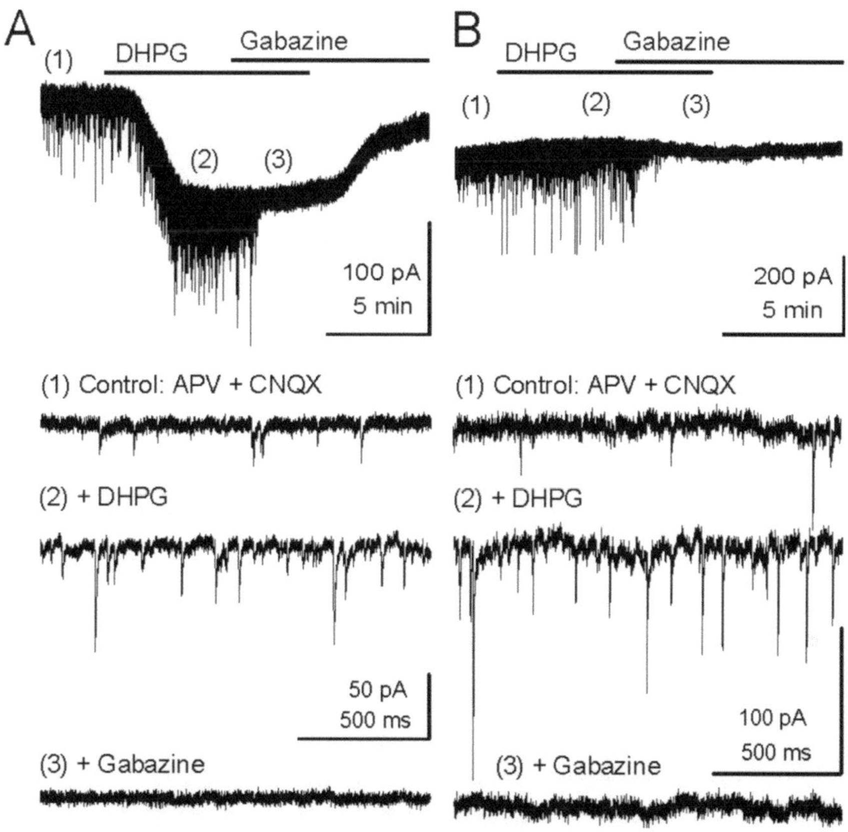

Fig. 6. DHPG increased the frequency of GABAergic IPSCs in mitral cells. Voltage clamp recordings from mitral cells were made with pipettes with a high chloride concentration during blockade of iGluRs. Under these conditions, chloride-mediated IPSCs are reversed in polarity and appear as downward deflections (inward currents). A: Upper trace - Application of mGluR agonist DHPG evoked an inward current in a mitral cell recorded in a slice from a wildtype mouse. Timepoints 1-3 are shown at faster timescale in the three lower tracers, respectively. Note the increase in frequency of fast IPSPs (trace 2), which are completely blocked by the $GABA_A$ receptor antagonist gabazine (trace 3). B: In a mitral cell from an mGluR1$^{-/-}$ mouse, the DHPG-evoked inward current was absent, but DHPG substantially increased the frequency of IPSCs. Recording conditions and labeling as in (A). From Heinbockel et al., 2007a with permission of The American Physiological Society.

the increase in IPSCs was accompanied by a large inward current (~-100 pA) in mitral cells, mediated by direct activation of mGluR1 (Heinbockel et al., 2004). To preclude mGluR1-mediated excitation of mitral cells, similar experiments were performed in mGluR1$^{-/-}$ mice. DHPG, applied in the presence of iGluR blockers, increased the frequency of IPSCs but did not elicit an inward current in mitral cells (Fig. 6B). IPSCs were abolished by the $GABA_A$ receptor antagonist gabazine (Fig. 6A, B).

2.7 Blockade of mGluRs reduces mitral cell-evoked excitation of granule cells and lateral inhibition in the MOB

Our results demonstrated that pharmacological activation of mGluRs increased GABAergic inhibition in the MOB. We hypothesized that functionally endogenous activation of mGluRs played a role in granule cell responses to glutamatergic synaptic input from mitral cells and that mGluRs are involved in granule cell-mediated feedback inhibition of mitral cells. Therefore, we assessed the effects of the mGluR antagonist LY341495 on granule cell responses to mitral cell input using optical imaging of a voltage sensitive dye (RH-414) (Heinbockel et al., 2007a). We used this imaging to investigate activity patterns evoked by stimulation of the lateral olfactory tract (LOT), the output tract for mitral/tufted cells to higher olfactory centers. By electrically stimulating the LOT, mitral cells can be activated directly. Mitral cells, in turn, activate mitral cell to granule cell glutamatergic synapses (Schoppa et al., 1998; Schoppa and Westbrook, 1999; Aroniadou-Anderjaska et al., 2000; Halabisky et al., 2000; Egger et al., 2005). Single electrical shocks applied to the LOT evoked optical responses that were first observed in the external plexiform layer (Laaris et al., 2007) and then spread sequentially into the

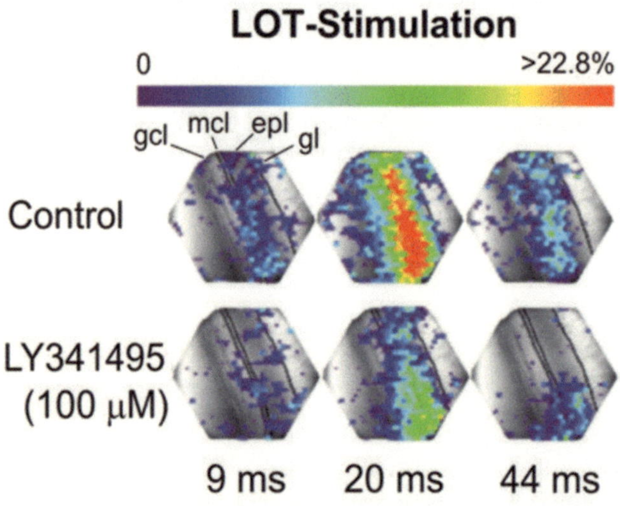

Fig. 7. mGluR antagonist LY341495 decreased temporal and spatial spread of evoked activity as revealed by voltage-sensitive dye imaging. Each panel shows the amplitude of optical responses, recorded by each of 464 photodiodes. Signal amplitudes, expressed as a percentage above mean baseline values, are color-coded; color scale at top applies to all images. Time intervals beneath the images are relative to the onset of LOT stimulation. Application of LY341495 reduced the amplitude of LOT-evoked optical signals. gl – glomerular layer; epl – external plexiform layer; mcl – mitral cell layer; gcl – granule cell layer; LOT – lateral olfactory tract. From Heinbockel et al., 2007a with permission of The American Physiological Society.

superficial granule cell layer. The LOT-evoked optical responses were abolished in calcium-free ACSF, by application of TTX or by washing-in of iGluR blockers (CNQX, APV), which indicated that the optical responses were mediated postsynaptically (Laaris et al., 2007). Application of the mGluR antagonist LY341495 reduced the peak amplitude of the LOT-evoked voltage-sensitive dye signal in the external plexiform layer by ~50% (Fig. 7) (Heinbockel et al., 2007a). Since the optical signals primarily reflect glutamatergic excitation of granule cell dendrites (Laaris et al., 2007), our findings suggest that mGluR blockade reduces granule cell excitability to mitral/tufted cell synaptic input. If mGluRs are pharmacologically inactivated, granule cells decrease their GABA release and this reduction in GABA release takes place in response to synaptic input from mitral/tufted cells.

3. Endocannabinoid signaling in the hippocampus

3.1 The endocannabinoid system

During the past decade, the endocannabinoid system has emerged as an important neuromodulatory system (Alger, 2002; Alger and Kim, 2011; Freund et al., 2003; Howlett et al., 2004), which involves cannabinoid receptors, CB1R, and their endogenous activators, the endocannabinoids (eCBs). CB1Rs are expressed at high levels in the brain (Herkenham et al., 1991; Matsuda et al., 1993), specifically at presynaptic nerve terminals (Katona et al., 1999; Tsou et al., 1999). Like the endogenous opiate system, the eCB system was first discovered because it can be activated by a plant-derived compound - in the case of the eCBs, this is Δ9-tetrahydrocannabinol, THC, the bioactive ingredient of the drugs marijuana and hashish (Ameri, 1999). Although artificially activated by the drug, eCB receptors exist in all normal brains (Herkenham et al., 1990, 1991; Matsuda et al., 1993) and subserve many essential brain functions when activated by their natural ligands. eCBs are the endogenous ligands for $G_{i/o}$-protein-coupled type 1 cannabinoid receptors (CB1 receptors, CB1Rs) and are synthesized from membrane lipids (DiMarzo et al., 1998). eCBs can diffuse through membranes and are thus able to activate receptors in the same manner as exogenous CBs. In the early 1990s, two eCBs were discovered (reviewed in Nicoll and Alger, 2003). These two eCBs, arachidonoylethanolamide (anandamide, AEA) and 2-arachidonoyl glycerol (2-AG), are produced in the brain, bind to CB1R and have the same functional activity as marijuana. The resemblance between marijuana and endocannabinoids allows marijuana to activate CB1R. However, it is the eCBs rather than marijuana that evolved together with CB1R to serve as a brain communication system.

Functionally, eCBs were found to mediate retrograde signals in the hippocampus (Maejima et al., 2001b; Ohno-Shosaku et al., 2001; Varma et al., 2001; Wilson and Nicoll, 2001; Wilson et al., 2001), cerebellum (Kreitzer and Regehr, 2001b; Maejima et al., 2001a; Yoshida et al., 2002), neocortex (Trettel and Levine, 2003, Trettel et al., 2004), and amygdala (Zhu and Lovinger, 2005; Kodirov et al., 2009). In contrast to conventional neurotransmitters, eCBs are fats, lipids and are not stored but rather are rapidly synthesized from components of the cell membrane. They are then released from places all over cells when levels of calcium rise inside the neuron or when certain G-protein-coupled receptors are activated. After release, eCBs bind to CB1Rs on nearby neurons and influence the ion channels on that neuron, e.g., through closure of those ion channels. For several years, eCBs played a mysterious role in the brain. Finally, eCBs were found to be responsible for a new type of neuronal communication, called DSI for depolarization-induced suppression of inhibition (Fig. 8) (reviewed in Alger, 2002; Nicoll and Alger, 2003). When the calcium concentration inside a

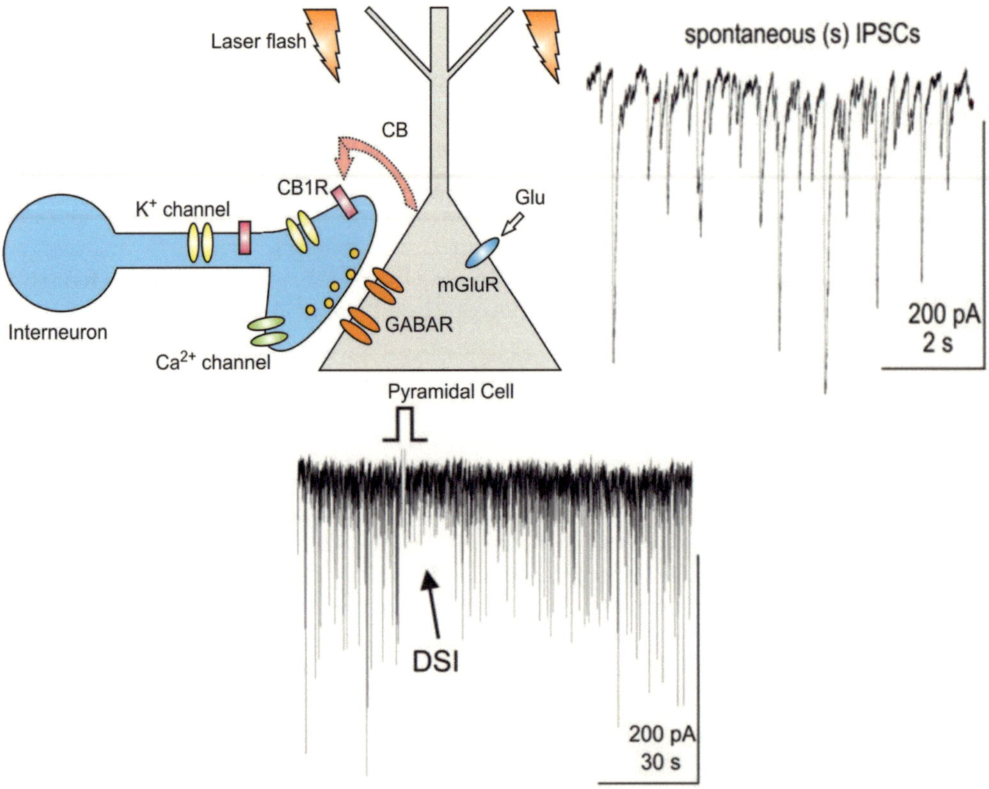

Fig. 8. Left panel: Depolarization-induced Suppression of Inhibition (DSI) is a model for retrograde signaling in the hippocampus and allows assaying real time release of eCBs from pyramidal cells as a brief cessation of GABA ouput. Activation of metabotropic glutamate receptors (mGluRs) on CA1 pyramidal neurons or depolarization of postsynaptic pyramidal cells evokes synthesis and release of cannabinoids (CBs). CBs bind to presynaptic CB receptors (CB1R) on GABAergic interneurons and transiently reduce GABA release from synaptic terminals. As a consequence, $GABA_A$ receptor-mediated synaptic currents and GABAergic inhibition are temporarily suppressed in pyramidal cells. Middle panel: Pyramidal cells shows spontaneous inhibitory postsynaptic currents (IPSCs). Right panel: In response to a 1-s voltage pulse the pyramidal cell reveals DSI, a transient reduction in IPSC activity as a result of endocannabinoids acting on CB1R on presynaptic GABAergic interneurons.

pyramidal cell of the hippocampus rises for a short time, incoming inhibitory signals in the form of GABA arriving from other neurons decline. The hypothesis was that during DSI, some unknown messenger must travel from the postsynaptic cell to the presynaptic GABA-releasing one and somehow turns off neurotransmitter release. When we think about signaling between nerve cells we most often refer to chemical synaptic signaling between two neurons, e.g., a GABAergic inhibitiory interneuron makes synaptic contacts with a pyramidal cell in the hippocampus. When the interneuron is activated it releases the inhibitory neurotransmitter GABA and inhibits the pyramidal cell. However, when the pyramidal cell is activated, e.g., through direct current injection, the inhibitory input onto the pyramidal cell is reduced. eCBs were found to act as retrograde signaling molecules that mediate communication between postsynaptic pyramidal cells and presynaptic inhibitory interneurons and evoke the reduction in GABA release. As fat-soluble molecules, eCBs do not diffuse over great distances in the watery extracellular environment of the brain. Thus, DSI acts as a short-lived local effect that enables individual neurons to disconnect briefly from their neighbors and encode information (Alger, 2002).

As summarized by Freund et al. (2003), eCBs evoke physiological responses, which may not be mediated by presynaptic CB1Rs but rather by postsynaptic CB1Rs, e.g., via regulation of K^+ conductances present on the extrasynaptic dendritic surface of neurons or modulation of postsynaptic NMDA receptors or even non-CB1R (e.g., Lozovaya et al., 2005). Furthermore, it is important to test the action of different CB1R ant-/agonists since several conventional CB1R ligands have been reported to have CB1R unspecific effects or activate non-CB1 receptors (Freund et al., 2003). For example, electrophysiological evidence suggests that the CB1R agonist WIN55,212-2 produces non-CB1R mediated effects on the excitability of principal neurons in the basolateral amygdala (Pistis et al., 2004), thus providing evidence for a non-CB1R site of action of WIN55,212-2 (Breivogel et al., 2001; Hajos et al., 2001).

The relevance of the eCB system for neural signaling and brain function in general has been explored only recently (Alger & Kim, 2011). A major advance came with the discovery that DSI, a type of short-term synaptic plasticity originally observed in the cerebellum and hippocampus, is mediated by eCBs (Alger, 2002; Freund et al., 2003). eCBs are retrograde signaling molecules that are released from depolarized principal neurons and travel to presynaptic inhibitory interneurons to reduce GABA release, a phenomenon known as depolarization-induced suppression of inhibition (DSI) (Fig. 8). DSI is a novel, regulatory process that is expressed as a transient suppression of synaptic $GABA_A$ responses mediated by retrograde signaling of eCBs from principal neurons. DSI can be used as a bioassay for real time release of eCBs from principal neurons (Alger, 2002; Heinbockel et al., 2005). Through the retrograde signaling process neurons alter the strength of synapses made onto them and thereby control their own synaptic excitability in an activity-dependent manner, which is functionally important in information processing by neuronal networks (Freund et al., 2003). In the cerebellum, a retrograde signaling process that is similar to DSI reduces synaptic excitation by suppressing presynaptic glutamate release and is called "DSE" (Kreitzer and Regehr, 2001a).

Our "classic" view of eCB action based on hippocampal studies is that eCBs reduce synaptic inhibition of the principal cell (DSI). eCBs were found to possess another property, namely, to mediate long-lasting self-inhibition in neocortical GABA-containing interneurons (Bacci et al., 2004). This self-inhibition is mediated by autocrine release of eCBs and does not depend on glutamatergic and/or GABAergic neurotransmission but rather on activity-dependent long-lasting hyperpolarization due to the activation of a K^+-conductance. eCBs released by these interneurons target the same cells and mediate a lasting hyperpolarization that is blocked by a CB1R antagonist. With self-inhibition cells can become hyperpolarized below spike threshold and are effectively removed from the neural circuit in which they reside.

The importance to understand the eCB system results from several general rationales: (1) An increasing body of knowledge exists about the relevance of eCBs in normal behaviors, including pain reception (Calignano et al., 1998) and feeding (Cota et al., 2003). (2) Research on the therapeutic potential of CBs has grown tremendously over the past few years (Iversen and Chapman, 2002). eCBs have been implicated in neuroprotection against acute excitotoxicity (Marsicano et al., 2003) and functional recovery after brain injury (Panikashvili et al., 2001). They regulate human airway function, which may provide a means for treatment of respiratory pathologies (Calignano et al., 2000). (3) Cannabinoids are in widespread use recreationally as psychoactive drugs and interact with other drugs of abuse, which emphasizes even more the need to understand the eCB system and the neurobiological substrate of their mood-altering capacity (Katona et al., 2001; Valjent et al., 2002), e.g., the eCB system is crucially involved in the extinction of aversive memories (Marsicano et al. 2002).

3.2 Photolysis and photoprobes

In electrophysiological experiments, traditionally the methodological approach to control synapses, cells or neural circuits has employed electrical stimulation with electrodes (Thompson et al., 2005). Electrodes generate local electrical fields that can trigger action potentials and lead to synaptic release of neurotransmitter. The use of electrodes allows for precise timing of stimulation but provides poor control over specificity and spatial extent of stimulation. As an alternative or additional experimental approach, chemical stimulation of synapses, cells, or circuits has been used by directly applying neurotransmitter or neuromodulators. However, these pharmacological approaches often yield little control of the stimulation in terms of timing, space and specificity. More recently, photo-uncaging of caged neurotransmitters has made the pharmacological approach more sophisticated. Photouncaging uses localized, patterned light and yields higher spatial and temporal resolution. Here, we foucs on one application of photostimulation, the flash photolysis technique, to determine signaling kinetics of the endocannabinoid system.

The endocannabinoid system constitutes a powerful tool for bioassaying the temporal dynamics or kinetics of lipid signaling (Heinbockel et al., 2005). Endocannabinoids are synthesized in, and released from, postsynaptic somatodendritic domains that are readily accessible to whole-cell patch electrodes. The dramatic effects of these lipid signals are detected electrophysiologically as CB1R-dependent alterations in conventional synaptic transmission, which therefore provide a sensitive means of bioassaying endocannabinoid levels and actions. Indeed, the first estimates of the speed of intercellular lipid signaling were provided by the study of DSI. Combining whole-cell voltage patch-clamp recording, intracellular calcium measurements, and photorelease of caged glutamate and a novel, caged cannabinoid, anandamide (AEA), we present data on signaling kinetics and describe the pivotal technological advances that allowed us to address this topic. Specifically, flash photolysis of caged compounds (photolysis using so-called molecular optical probes or photoprobes) was an important tool in these experiments. Caged compounds are inert, biologically inactive (e.g., a caged cannabinoid or caged glutamate) until a flash of laser light breaks open the molecular cage, releases the caged molecule and generates a biologically active effector molecule in situ (Kao, 2008). Chemically, the caged compound is a modified signal molecule. The modification of the molecule prevents its bioactivity until light absorption results in a photochemical change of the signal molecule such that its bioactivity is restored. Principally, the photochemically generated molecule can be a receptor agonist or antagonist which allows the experimenter to switch biological processes either on or off. Photolysis provides a means to control biological processes with light and to investigate these processes both temporally and spatially within living cells at the subcellular level (Thompson et al., 2005). Beside caged compounds, photoprobes also comprise fluorescent indicators (Kao, 2008). These indicators are molecules that change their fluorescent properties in response to a change in the physical or chemical environment. Known fluorescent indicators include calcium indicators or membrane potential indicators.

Kao (2008) points out three distinct advantages of photolysis of caged molecules over conventional techniques of molecule delivery: (1) temporal resolution, (2) spatial resolution, and (3) control over chemical identity of the signal molecule. In our studies of hippocampal cannabinoid signaling (Heinbockel et al., 2005), we pre-equilibrated the tissue with the biologically inactive caged molecules (caged anandamide or caged glutamate) before experimentation. During the experiment, a flash of laser light rapidly generated the biologically active signal molecules in situ. The released molecules were able to immediately interact with the receptors. The classic problems that can occur during bath application of drugs such as mixing, diffusion and access to receptors in brain slices are minimal. The photorelease of caged molecules can occur within a few microseconds to about 1 millisecond and, thus, allows for manipulation of the neurophysiology in the same time range. In addition to the temporal precision of drug delivery, photolysis affords high spatial resolution in the range of 0.5 micrometers. The laser light beam can easily be manipulated in space and focused on a small target, e.g., a dendrite. Kao (2008) describes the diffraction-limited spot with a diameter $d = 1.22\lambda/NA$. λ is the wavelength of light used which is typically UV light near 350 nm. NA is the numerical aperture of the focusing lens which is less than 1.0 in our case. This brings the resolution to better than 0.5 µm. Biological signaling molecules can be chemically or enzymatically labile. Ideally, uncaging of molecules generates stable molecules that are not easily broken down in the tissue or cell. In this case, flash photolysis generates authentic bioactive molecules in situ and provides a means to have precise control not only over temporal and spatial resolution of molecule delivery but also over the chemical identity of the delivered molecules.

3.3 Kinetics of lipid signaling

In contrast to classic neurotransmitters, eCBs are lipids and not stored but rather rapidly synthesized from components of the cell membrane. Mobilization of eCBs can occur through Ca^{2+}-dependent or relatively Ca^{2+}-independent pathways, with different down-stream effects. eCBs are released from places all over cells when levels of calcium rise inside the neuron or when certain G-protein-coupled receptors are activated.

After release from the cell, eCBs bind to CB1R on nearby neurons and cause a reversible, short-term depression of synaptic transmission, DSI (Fig. 8). In DSI, the excitation of a hippocampal CA1 pyramidal neuron leads to a transient reduction of GABA release from presynaptic terminals of inhibitory interneurons. Until now, insights into eCB action have been derived primarily from pharmacological experiments, because the intrinsic properties of eCBs have hampered direct physiological study of eCB signaling at CNS synapses (Heinbockel et al., 2005). The hydrophobicity of eCBs severely limits their penetration into brain tissue, and eCBs are rapidly degraded by abundant endogenous lipases. To circumvent these obstacles, our collaborator Joe Kao designed a highly water-soluble caged anandamide that is inert to lipases. When perfused into hippocampal slice preparations, the caged anandamide serves as a latent eCB pool, and focal photolysis rapidly liberates highly hydrophobic anandamide *in situ* to activate CB1R.

The eCB system constitutes a powerful tool for bioassaying the temporal dynamics of lipid signaling, the kinetics of lipid signaling. eCBs are synthesized in, and released from hippocampal pyramidal cells that are readily accessible to whole-cell patch clamp electrodes. The effects of eCBs are detected electrophysiologically as cannabinoid-dependent changes in conventional synaptic transmission between GABAergic, inhibitory interneurons and the recorded pyramidal cell, which therefore provide a sensitive means of bioassaying eCB levels. With DSI as an electrophysiological bioassay, we have used whole-cell voltage-clamp recording and intracellular Ca^{2+} measurement in combination with photorelease of caged anandamide and caged glutamate to probe the dynamics of the eCB signaling system in the CA1 region of rat cultured hippocampal slices (Heinbockel et al., 2005). Organotypic hippocampal slice cultures were prepared either as roller-tube cultures (Gähwiler et al., 1998) or as interface cultures on semiporous membranes (Stoppini et al., 1991). This type of brain slice thins out during the culturing process compared to acute slices and, therefore, allows light and drugs to easily penetrate the few cell layers of the cultured slice.

Fig. 8 shows a patch-clamp recording from a hippocampal pyramidal cell to illustrate the spontaneous inhibitory currents, sIPSCs and how they are transiently dampened by a voltage pulse applied to the pyramidal cell. Activation of the pyramidal cell results in a reduction of its inhibitory synaptic input. This experiment also allowed us to estimate the latency from the start of the voltage pulse to the onset of DSI which is around 350 to 400 ms (Fig. 9).

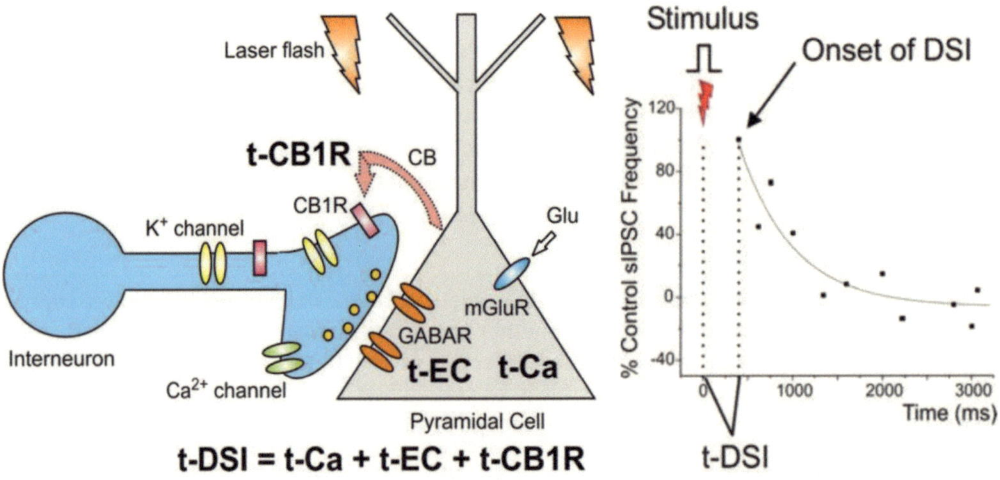

Fig. 9. Left panel: Diagram illustrating the different components that contribute to the onset latency of DSI after the initial stimulation (left panel). Right panel: Diagram illustrating the measurement of t-DSI, the latency from the time of stimulation (voltage step) to the start of DSI (onset of DSI).

The temporal dynamics of the lipid signaling pathway comprises several temporal components that we need to determine to quantify the time that it takes from the DSI-inducing stimulus to the onset of DSI. We ask what contributes to the latency to onset of DSI (start of DSI-inducing stimulus to initial suppression of IPSCs). Among these factors is the rise of calcium to initiate eCB synthesis (t-Ca) (Fig. 9). The rise in intracellular calcium leads to eCB synthesis and release of eCBs followed by travel of eCBs to CB1R on presynaptic interneurons, t-EC. The next step is the activation of CB1R and downstream effects, t-CB1R.

Time-to-onset of DSI (t-DSI):

- Rise of calcium to initiate CB synthesis, t-Ca
- CB synthesis, release, and travel to CB1R, t-EC
- Activation of CB1R and downstream steps, t-CB1R

t-DSI = t-Ca + t-EC + t-CB1R

We had available a novel caged form of anandamide (AEA), that is biologically inert and highly hydrophilic, such that it can easily reach its target in the slice preparation. A flash of UV laser light breaks open the cage and releases the cannabinoid, i.e., anandamide, which can bind immediately to its receptor (Fig. 10). Our experiments revealed that photorelease of anandamide suppressed sIPSCs. It took about 180 ms from the laser flash to the reduction of inhibitory currents detected with our patch clamp electrode in the pyramidal cell (Fig. 10). This experiment revealed that t-CB1R is ~180ms, i.e., direct activation of CB1R by photoreleasing anandamide results in suppression of sIPSCs in ~180ms. Photorelease of anandamide transiently suppressed spontaneous IPSCs with a time course comparable with that of DSI in Fig. 8, supporting the role of eCBs as mediator of the process.

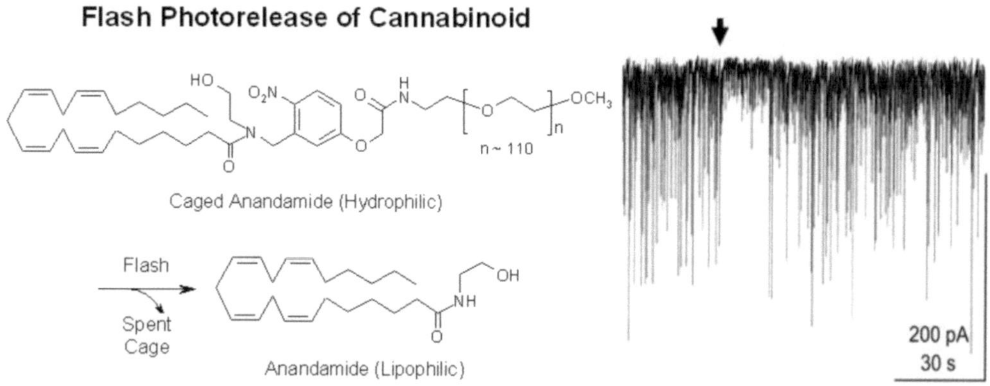

Fig. 10. Left panel: Photolysis of caged anandamide yields bioactive anandamide. Right panel: Photorelease of anandamide suppresses sIPSCs after a delay of ~180 ms. Modified from Heinbockel et al., 2005 with permission of the Society for Neuroscience.

The specifics of the photolysis and laser set-up were as follows (from Heinbockel et al., 2005): photorelease is expected to be complete in <100 µs, quantum efficiency for photorelease of AEA on photolysis is 0.062. The concentration of AEA was 200 µM. A multiline UV emission of an argon ion laser (wavelength, 333-364 nm; BeamLok 2065-7S; Spectra Physics) was launched into a 100 µm diameter fused silica optical fiber (OZ Optics). The exit end of the fiber was projected onto a conjugate of the field diaphragm plane along the epifluorescence path of the microscope. Once we established a whole-cell recording from a CA1 pyramidal cell, the laser spot (~15-20 µm diameter) was centered on the soma of the patched cell. Output from the laser was controlled by a shutter (NM Laser Products, Sunnyvale, CA) to generate photolytic flashes (100 ms duration). In our experimental setup, an instrumentation delay of 1.4 ms occurred from triggering the UV laser flash to a laser signal measured by the photomultiplier (PMT).

For our recordings we used an Axoclamp 2B amplifier and a Digidata-1200A Interface (Molecular Devices - Axon Instruments, Union City, CA). Analog signals were recorded, digitized at 5kHz, low-pass filtered at 2 kHz, and subsequently analyzed using Clampfit (Clampfit 9, Axon Instruments) and Mini Analysis Program (version 6.0.1. Synaptosoft Inc., Decatur, GA). Fig. 11 illustrates the averaged data for photolysis-induced suppression of inhibition (PSI) evoked by photorelease of anandamide in the absence or presence of a specific CB1R antagonist, AM251. The antagonist prevented the effect of photoreleased anandamide and demonstrated that DSI occurred as a result of uncaging anandamide.

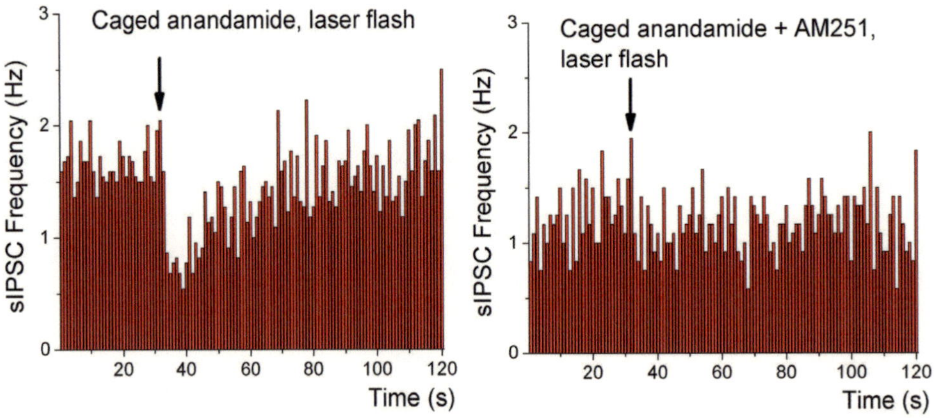

Fig. 11. Left panel: Dynamics of spontaneous IPSC suppression by photorelease of anandamide in cultured hippocampal slices. Photorelease of caged anandamide, present at 200 μM, by a 100 ms UV laser flash (arrow) transiently suppressed spontaneous IPSCs (downward deflections) recorded under whole-cell voltage clamp from a CA1 pyramidal cell at room temperature with ionotropic glutamate receptors blocked. Right panel: The selective CB1R antagonist AM251 blocked anandamide-evoked PSI (photolysis induced suppression of inhibition). Arrow indicates laser flash. Modified from Heinbockel et al., 2005 with permission of the Society for Neuroscience.

3.4 Calcium dependence of depolarization-induced suppression of inhibition

The two major eCBs, anandamide and 2-arachidonoyl glycerol, are both derivatives of arachidonic acid (Iversen, 2003; Freund et al., 2003, for review) and are agonists at CB1R. Both AEA and 2-AG can be released from postsynaptic principal cell somata and dendrites, and their release is stimulated by a marked rise in $[Ca^{2+}]_i$. Therefore, we determined the calcium dependence of DSI by using voltage pulses of different duration while measuring intracellular calcium with a calcium indicator (fluo-3 with a PMT).

Ca^{2+}-dependent fluo-3 (50 μM in the whole-cell pipette) fluorescence was collected by a photomultiplier tube (PMT) (H5783, Hamamatsu) and recorded concurrently with IPSCs. A filter set suitable for fluo-3 (Chroma 41025, exciter HQ470/40x, emitter HQ515/30m, dichroic Q495LP) was used in conjunction with a Nikon Eclipse 600 upright microscope (40x objective). The output of the PMT was low-pass filtered at 2 kHz (Frequency Devices), sent to a Digidata 1322, digitized at 5 kHz and displayed by pClamp9 (Axon Instruments) using Clampex. Trials were analyzed off-line using Origin software (OriginPro 7, OriginLab Corp, Northampton, MA). To correct fluorescence baseline drift caused by gradual photobleaching, two 3-sec segments (immediately before photolytic or electrical stimulation, and at the end of each fluorescence record) were fit by a single exponential, which was used as the baseline. Our experiments revealed that it took about 60 ms to evoke a calcium transient sufficient for minimal DSI, i.e., for intracellular calcium to rise and evoke eCB synthesis and release (Fig. 12).

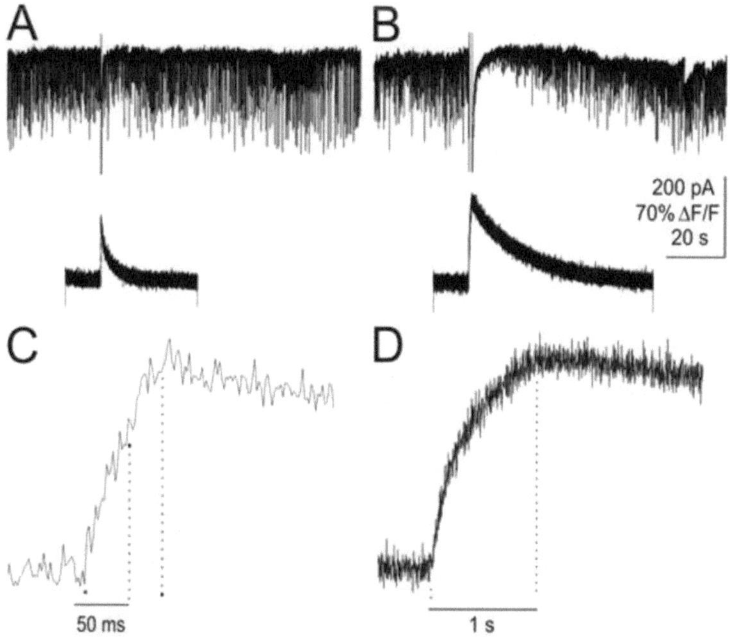

Fig. 12. Calcium dependence of DSI. A: A 50 ms voltage step resulted in minimal DSI in a pyramidal cell. In this neuron, the sIPSC frequency before the voltage step was 6.65 Hz (averaged over 32 s before the step) and 5.55 Hz after the step (averaged over 20 s after the step). This represents a 16.6% reduction in sIPSC frequency. The accompanying Ca^{2+} transient (fluo-3 signal) was measured with a PMT and is shown immediately below and, on a faster time scale, in C. The peak of the transient occurred after the end of the voltage step. B: A 1 s voltage step evoked pronounced DSI. The frequency before the step was 6.43 Hz and was reduced to 1.75 Hz after the step (averaged over 20 s after the step) (i.e., a 72.8% reduction in sIPSC frequency). The Ca^{2+} signal for the 1 s step was substantially larger than in A and peaked at the end of the voltage step (D). Ca^{2+} transients in C and D were normalized to facilitate visual comparison. The dotted lines in C mark the terminations of the 50 ms voltage step and peak of the Ca^{2+} transient (determined from the trace after a smoothing procedure). In D, the dotted line shows that the peak of the Ca^{2+} transient occurred at the end of the 1 s voltage step. From Heinbockel et al., 2005 with permission of the Society for Neuroscience.

These experiments allowed us to determine the time for synthesis and release of eCB from the postsynaptic neuron, which was estimated to be around 150 ms at room temperature, comparable with the timescale of metabotropic signaling and at least an order of magnitude faster than previously thought. A major portion of the DSI onset time, t-DSI, reflected activation of presynaptic CB1Rs and downstream consequences. These findings suggest that, far from simply serving long-term neuromodulatory functions, eCB signaling is sufficiently fast to exert moment-to-moment control of synaptic transmission.

- t-DSI = t-Ca + t-EC + t-CB1R
- t-DSI, onset latency: 350 to 400 ms after voltage step
- t-CB1R: direct activation of CB1R by photoreleasing anandamide results in suppression of sIPSCs in ~180ms
- t-Ca: 50-ms voltage step evokes a calcium transient sufficient to obtain minimal DSI (t-Ca: ~60 ms)
- t-EC: ~150 ms for eCB synthesis and release to occur

3.5 Dynamics of mGluR-dependent endocannabinoid suppression of sIPSCs

Activation of several G-protein coupled receptors (GPCRs) can trigger the release of eCBs for many minutes, e.g., dopamine (Giuffrida et al., 1999), metabotropic glutamate (Maejima et al., 2001a; Varma et al., 2001; Ohno-Shosaku et al., 2002) or muscarinic acetylcholine receptors (Kim et al., 2002; Ohno-Shosaku et al., 2003). eCBs are typically released in a calcium-dependent manner (Di Marzo et al., 1994; Stella et al., 1997). In the mGluR- and mAChR-dependent pathways no clear rise in intracellular calcium $[Ca^{2+}]_i$ (Maejima et al., 2001a; Kim et al., 2002) is necessary. Release of eCBs can be triggered even in the presence of high intracellular concentrations of calcium chelators, although they may nevertheless be sensitive to ambient $[Ca^{2+}]_i$ (Hashimotodani et al., 2005). We asked if these pathways function on the same time scale as voltage-activated DSI.

Therefore, we determined the dynamic components of the mGluR-induced eCB response on sIPSC frequency in pyramidal cells (Fig. 13). The mean onset latency, duration and magnitude of the IPSC suppression caused by uncaged glutamate were similar to that caused by uncaged AEA (Figs. 9, 10). No reduction in sIPSCs occurred for 221 ms (determined by extrapolation of the exponential fit to the control sIPSC level). If the time-to-onset of IPSC suppression caused by the mGluR-induced eCB process (time to mGluR-dependent suppression of inhibition, $t_{mGluRSI}$) is described by: t-mGluR-SI = 221 ms = t-eCB(mGluR) + t-CB1R, where t-eCB(mGluR) is the time for activation of the mGluR-dependent eCB synthesis and release, and t-CB1R is ~180 ms (see above), then t-eCB(mGluR) would be < 50 ms. This is even faster than eCB synthesis and released evoked by a voltage step.

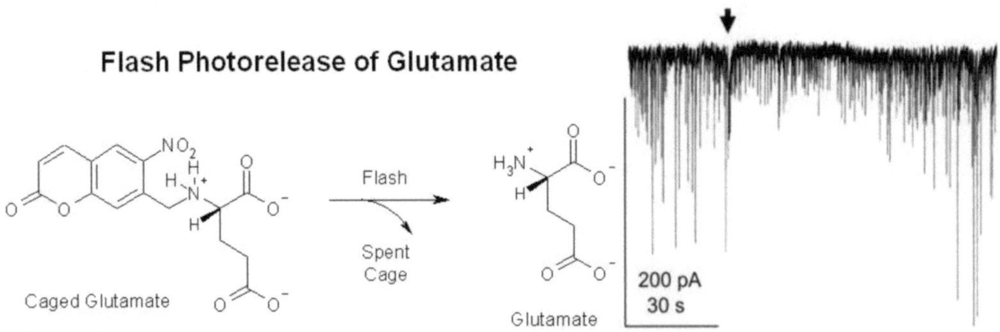

Fig. 13. Dynamics of mGluR-dependent endocannabinoid suppression of sIPSCs in cultured hippocampal slices. Left panel: Photorelease of glutamate. Right panel: Recording from a pyramidal cell illustrates the transient reduction in spontaneous (s) IPSC frequency of CA1 pyramidal cells after flash photorelease of caged glutamate (photolysis induced suppression of inhibition, PSI). Arrow indicates laser flash. From Heinbockel et al., 2005 with permission of the Society for Neuroscience.

4. Conclusion

mGluR1 in mitral cells and mGluR5 in granule cells are expressed in higher density in the MOB than in most other regions of the brain suggesting a critical functional role for mGluRs in the operations of the MOB network. We described new findings demonstrating that the excitability of mitral cells and granule cells is directly and potently modulated via activation of mGluRs by endogenously released glutamate in MOB slices. Our findings indicate that the net effect of the mGluR actions is to increase mitral cell excitatory drive on granule cells, and in turn, to increase GABA release from granule cells. A combination of patch clamp recording and voltage-sensitive dye imaging experiments suggest that a major functional consequence of mGluR activation is to increase both the spatial spread and temporal duration of lateral inhibition in the MOB. Potentially, at the network level, mGluRs in the MOB function to increase contrast for odorant-induced activity patterns.

The speed with which neuromodulators act places critical constraints on the physiological roles they can play and yet there was no detailed information regarding the dynamics of eCB effects. In order to investigate this issue, we developed an optical tool – a photolytically 'caged' form of one of the principal eCBs, anandamide. Release of anandamide from its caged form by a UV-laser flash rapidly activated presynaptic CB1Rs and suppressed the release of GABA (Heinbockel et al., 2005). We also showed that a specific CB1R antagonist, AM 251, blocked the suppression of spontaneous IPSCs. We have therefore established that uncaged anandamide can be used as a CB1R agonist to study activation of CB1R in the brain. Similarly, uncaged glutamate acted at mGluRs on hippocampal pyramidal cells to evoke CB release and subsequent suppression of presynaptic GABA release (Heinbockel et al., 2005). We provide the first detailed attempt to determine the minimal time required for activation of an intercellular neuronal lipid messenger system. A major portion of DSI onset time, t-DSI, reflects activation of presynaptic CB1R and downstream consequences. eCBs, and by extension similar lipid messengers, can be mobilized and evoke responses as quickly as conventional metabotropic, GPCR-coupled neurotransmitters. The role of lipids in brain signaling is not relegated to homeostatic processes or slowly-activating forms of regulation, but rather lipids can affect neuronal excitability in moment-to-moment information processing. Light can be used as a tool for manipulating biological structures and events. The experimental approach described represents technology that has wide application in neurobiology. This powerful new technology will invariably stimulate new types of experiments.

5. Acknowledgment

This work was supported in part by the Whitehall Foundation, National Institutes of Health National Institute of General Medical Sciences (S06GM08016) and National Institutes of Health National Institute of Neurological Disorders and Stroke (U54NS039407). I am grateful to Dr. Philip M. Heyward, Dunedin, New Zealand for his initial input to this chapter and to Dr. Adam Puche, Baltimore, MD, for technical assistance with confocal microscopy. I would like to gratefully acknowledge Drs. Bradley E. Alger, Matthew Ennis, and Joseph P. Y. Kao.

6. References

Alger BE (2002) Retrograde signaling in the regulation of synaptic transmission: focus on endocannabinoids. Progress in Neurobiology 68:247-286. ISSN 0301- 0082

Alger BE, Kim J (2011) Supply and demand for endocannabinoids. Trends in Neurosciences 34:304-315. ISSN: 0166- 2236

Ameri A (1999) The effects of cannabinoids on the brain. Progress in Neurobiology 58:315-348. ISSN 0301- 0082

Aroniadou-Anderjaska V, Ennis M, Shipley MT (1997) Glomerular synaptic responses to olfactory nerve input in rat olfactory bulb slices. Neuroscience 79:425-34. ISSN 0306-4522

Aroniadou-Anderjaska V, Ennis M, Shipley MT (1999). Current-source density analysis in the rat olfactory bulb: laminar distribution of kainate/AMPA and NMDA receptor-mediated currents. Journal of Neurophysiology 81:15-28. ISSN 0022-3077

Aroniadou-Anderjaska, V., Zhou, F.-M., Priest, C.A., Ennis, M., and Shipley, M.T. (2000). GABA-B receptor-mediated presynaptic inhibition of sensory input to the olfactory bulb. Journal of Neurophysiology 84:1194-1203. ISSN 0022-3077

Bacci A, Huguenard JR, Prince DA (2004) Long-lasting self-inhibition of neocortical interneurons mediated by endocannabinoids. Nature 431:312-316. ISSN 0028-0836

Balu, R., Pressler, R.T., & Strowbridge, B.W. (2007) Multiple modes of synaptic excitation of olfactory bulb granule cells. Journal of Neuroscience 27:5621-32. ISSN 0270-6474

Breivogel CS, Griffin G, Di Marzo V, Martin BR (2001) Evidence for a new G protein-coupled cannabinoid receptor in mouse brain. Molecular Pharmacology 60:155-63. ISSN 0026-895X

Calignano A, La Rana G, Giuffrida A, Piomelli D (1998) Control of pain initiation by endogenous cannabinoids. Nature 394:277-281. ISSN 0028-0836

Calignano A, Katona I, Desarnaud F, Giuffrida A, La Rana G, Mackie K, Freund TF, Piomelli D (2000) Bidirectional control of airway responsiveness by endogenous cannabinoids. Nature 408:96-101. ISSN 0028-0836

Chiamulera, C., Epping-Jordan, M.P., Zocchi, A., Marcon, C., Cottiny, C., Tacconi, S., Corsi, M., Orzi, F., and Conquet, F. (2001). Reinforcing and locomotor stimulant effects of cocaine are absent in mGluR5 null mutant mice. Nature Neuroscience 4:873-874. ISSN 1097-6256

Clark, B.P., Baker, S.R., Goldsworthy, J., Harris, J.R., and Kingston, A.E. (1997). 2-Methyl-4-carboxyphenylglycine (LY367385) selectively antagonizes metabotropic glutamate mGluR1 receptors. Bioorganic & Medicinal Chemistry Letters 7:2777-2870. ISSN: 0960-894X

Conquet, F., Bashir, Z.I., Davies, C.H., Daniel, H., Ferraguti, F., Bordi, F., Franz-Bacon, K., Reggiani, A., Matarese, V., Condé, F., Collingridge, G.L., and Crépel, F. (1994). Motor deficit and impairment of synaptic plasticity in mice lacking mGluR1. Nature 372:237-243. ISSN 0028-0836

Conn PJ, Pin JP (1997) Pharmacology and functions of metabotropic glutamate receptors. Annual Review of Pharmacology and Toxicology 37:205-237. ISSN 0362-1642

Cota D, Marsicano G, Lutz B, Vicennati V, Stalla GK, Pasquali R, Pagotto (2003) Endogenous cannabinoid system as a modulator of food intake. International Journal of Obesity 27:289-301. ISSN 0307-0565

Di Marzo V, Fontana A, Cadas H, Schinelli S, Cimino G, Schwartz JC, Piomelli D (1994) Formation and inactivation of endogenous cannabinoid anandamide in central neurons. Nature 372:686-691. ISSN 0028-0836

Diana MA, Levenes C, Mackie K, Marty A (2002) Short-term retrograde inhibition of GABAergic synaptic currents in rat Purkinje cells is mediated by endogenous cannabinoids. Journal of Neuroscience 22:200-208. ISSN 0270-6474

Dingledine, R., Borges, K., Bowie, D., & Traynellis, S.F. (1999). The glutamate receptor ion channels. Pharmacological Reviews, 51:7-61. ISSN 0031-6997

Dong HW, Heinbockel T, Hamilton KA, Hayar A, Ennis M (2009) Metabotropic glutamate receptors and dendrodendritic synapses in the main olfactory bulb. Annals of the New York Academy of Sciences 1170: 224-238 ISSN 0077-8923

Egger, V., Svoboda, K., and Mainen, Z.F. (2005). Dendrodendritic synaptic signals in olfactory bulb granule cells: local spine boost and global low-threshold spike. Journal of Neuroscience 25: 3521-3530. ISSN 0270-6474

Ennis M, Hayar A, Hamilton KA (2007) Neurochemistry of the main olfactory system. In: Handbook of Neurochemistry and Molecular Neurobiology (edited by Lajtha A), Sensory Neurochemistry, edited by Johnson DA. Springer: Heidelberg. 137-204. ISBN 978-0-387-35478-1

Freund TF, Katona I, Piomelli D (2003) Role of endogenous cannabinoids in synaptic signaling. Physiological Reviews 83:1017-1066. ISSN: 0031-9333

Giuffrida A, Parsons LH, Kerr TM, Rodriguez de Fonseca F, Navarro M, Piomelli D (1999) Dopamine activation of endogenous cannabinoid signaling in dorsal striatum. Nature Neuroscience 2:358-363. ISSN 1097-6256

Hajos N, Ledent C, Freund TF (2001) Novel cannabinoid-sensitive receptor mediates inhibition of glutamatergic synaptic transmission in the hippocampus. Neuroscience 106:1-4. ISSN 0306-4522

Halabisky, B., Friedman, D., Radojicic, M., and Strowbridge, B. (2000). Calcium influx through NMDA receptors directly evokes GABA release in olfactory bulb granule cells. Journal of Neuroscience 20:5124-5134. ISSN 0270-6474

Hashimotodani Y, Ohno-Shosaku T, Tsubokawa H, Ogata H, Emoto K, Maejima T, Araishi K, Shin HS, Kano M (2005) Phospholipase C_{β} serves as a coincidence detector through its Ca^{2+} dependency for triggering retrograde endocannabinoid signal. Neuron 45:257-268. ISSN 0896-6273

Heinbockel T, Heyward P, Conquet F, Ennis M (2004) Regulation of main olfactory bulb mitral cell excitability by metabotropic glutamate receptor mGluR1. Journal of Neurophysiology 92: 3085-3096. ISSN 0022-3077

Heinbockel T, Brager DH, Reich C, Zhao J, Muralidharan S, Alger BE, Kao JPY (2005) Endocannabinoid signaling dynamics probed with optical tools. Journal of Neuroscience 25: 9449-9459. ISSN 0270-6474

Heinbockel T, Laaris N, Ennis M (2007a) Metabotropic glutamate receptors in the main olfactory bulb drive granule cell-mediated inhibition. Journal of Neurophysiology 97: 858-870. ISSN 0022-3077

Heinbockel T, Hamilton KA, Ennis M (2007b) Group I metabotropic glutamate receptors are differentially expressed by two populations of olfactory bulb granule cells. Journal of Neurophysiology 97: 3136-3141. ISSN 0022-3077

Heinbockel T, Ennis M (2008) Metabotropic glutamate receptors and neural processing in the olfactory system. In: Neural Pathways Research. Pichler FL (ed), Nova Science Publishers, New York, chapter 1, pp. 1-30. ISBN 1-60456-214-5

Heinbockel T, Heyward PM (2009) Glutamate synapses in olfactory neural circuits. In: Amino Acid Receptor Research. Paley BF, Warfield TE (eds), Nova Science Publishers, New York, chapter 16, pp. 379-414. ISBN 1-60456-283-8

Herkenham M, Lynn AB, Little MD, Johnson MR, Melvin LS, de Costa BR, Rice KC (1990) Cannabinoid receptor localization in brain. Proceedings of the National Academcy of Sciences USA 87:1932–1936. ISSN 0027-8424

Herkenham M, Lynn AB, Johnson MR, Melvin LS, de Costa BR, Rice KC (1991) Characterization and localization of cannabinoid receptors in rat brain: a quantitative in vitro autoradiographic study. Journal of Neuroscience 11:563-583. ISSN 0270-6474

Hoffman AF, Lupica CR (2000) Mechanisms of cannabinoid inhibition of GABA(A) synaptic transmission in the hippocampus. Journal of Neuroscience 20:2470-2479. ISSN 0270-6474

Howlett AC, Breivogel CS, Childers SR, Deadwyler SA, Hampson RE, Porrino LJ (2004) Cannabinoid physiology and pharmacology: 30 years of progress. Neuropharmacology 47:345-358. ISSN 0028-3908

Iversen L, Chapman V (2002) Cannabinoids: a real prospect for pain relief. Current Opinion in Pharmacology 2:50-55

Iversen L (2003) Cannabis and the brain. Brain 126:1252-70. ISSN 0006-8950

Kao JPY (2008) Controlling neurophysiology with light and caged molecules. In: Optical control of neural excitability. (Keshishian H, ed) pp. 1-12. Washington, DC: Society for Neuroscience.

Katona I, Sperlagh B, Sik A, Kafalvi A, Vizi ES, Mackie K, Freund TF (1999) Presynaptically located CB1 cannabinoid receptors regulate GABA release from axon terminals of specific hippocampal interneurons. Journal of Neuroscience 19:4544-4558. ISSN 0270-6474

Katona I, Rancz EA, Acsady L, Ledent C, Mackie K, Hajos N, Freund TF (2001) Distribution of CB1 cannabinoid receptors in the amygdala and their role in the control of GABAergic transmission. Journal of Neuroscience 21:9506-9518. ISSN 0270-6474

Keller A, Yagodin S, Aroniadou-Anderjaska A, Zimmer LA, Ennis M, Sheppard NF, Shipley MT (1998) Functional organization of rat olfactory bulb glomeruli revealed by optical imaging. Journal of Neuroscience 18:2602-2612. ISSN 0270-6474

Kim J, Isokawa M, Ledent C, Alger BE (2002) Activation of muscarinic acetylcholine receptors enhances the release of endogenous cannabinoids in the hippocampus. Journal of Neuroscience 22:10182-10191. ISSN 0270-6474

Kinoshita A, Shigemoto R, Ohishi H, van der Putten H, Mizuno N (1998) Immunohistochemical localization of metabotropic glutamate receptors, mGluR7a and mGluR7b, in the central nervous system of the adult rat and mouse: a light and electron microscopic study. Journal of Comparative Neurology 393:332-52. ISSN 1096-9861

Kinzie JM, Saugstad JA, Westbrook GL, Segerson TP (1995) Distribution of metabotropic glutamate receptor 7 messenger RNA in the developing and adult rat brain. Neuroscience 69:167-76. ISSN 0306-4522

Kodirov SA, Jasiewicz J, Amirmahani P, Psyrakis D, Bonni K, Wehrmeister M, Lutz B (2009) Endogenous cannabinoids trigger the depolarization-induced suppression of excitation in the lateral amygdala. Learning & Memory 17:43-49. ISSN 1072-0502

Kreitzer AC, Regehr WG (2001a) Retrograde inhibition of presynaptic calcium influx by endogenous cannabinoids at excitatory synapses onto Purkinje cells. Neuron 29:717-727. ISSN 0896-6273

Kreitzer AC, Regehr WG (2001b) Cerebellar depolarization-induced suppression of inhibition is mediated by endogenous cannabinoids. Journal of Neuroscience 21:RC174. ISSN 0270-6474

Laaris, N., Puche, A., and Ennis, M. (2007). Complementary postsynaptic activity patterns elicited in olfactory bulb by stimulation of mitral/tufted and centrifugal fiber inputs to granule cells. Journal of Neurophysiology 97:296-306. ISSN 0022-3077

Lea, P.M., and Faden, A.I. (2003) Modulation of metabotropic glutamate receptors as potential treatment for acute and chronic neurodegenerative disorders. Drug News & Perspectives 16:513-22. ISSN 0214-0934

Levenes C, Daniel H, Soubrie P, Crepel F (1998) Cannabinoids decrease excitatory synaptic transmission and impair long-term depression in rat cerebellar Purkinje cells. Journal of Physiology (Lond) 510:867-879. ISSN 0022-3751

Liu, W.-L., and Shipley, M.T. (1994) Cholecystokinin (CCK) immunocytochemical characteristics and postsynaptic targets of the intrabulbar associational system in the rat olfactory bulb. Journal of Comparative Neurology 346:541-558. ISSN 1096-9861

Lozovaya N, Yatsenko N, Beketov A, Tsintsadze T, Burnashev N (2005) Glycine receptors in CNS neurons as a target for nonretrograde action of cannabinoids. Journal of Neuroscience 25:7499-7506. ISSN 0270-6474

Maejima T, Hashimoto K, Yoshida T, Aiba A, Kano M (2001a) Presynaptic inhibition caused by retrograde signal from metabotropic glutamate to cannabinoid receptors. Neuron 31:463-475. ISSN 0896-6273

Maejima T, Ohno-Shosaku T, Kano M (2001b) Endogenous cannabinoid as a retrograde messenger from depolarized postsynaptic neurons to presynaptic terminals. Neuroscience Research 40:205-210. ISSN 0168-0102

Marsicano G, Wotjak CT, Azad SC, Bisogno T, Rammes G, Cascio MG, Hermann H, Tang J, Hofmann C, Zieglgansberger W, Di Marzo V, Lutz B (2002) The endogenous cannabinoid system controls extinction of aversive memories. Nature 418:530-534. ISSN 0028-0836

Marsicano G, Goodenough S, Monory K, Hermann H, Eder M, Cannich A, Azad SC, Cascio MG, Gutierrez SO, van der Stelt M, Lopez-Rodriguez ML, Casanova E, Schutz G, Zieglgansberger W, Di Marzo V, Behl C, Lutz B (2003) CB1 cannabinoid receptors and on-demand defense against excitotoxicity. Science 302:84-88. ISSN 0036-8075

Martin LJ, Blackstone CD, Huganir RL, Price DL (1992) Cellular localization of a metabotropic glutamate receptor in rat brain. Neuron 9:259-270. ISSN 0896-6273

Masu M, Tanabe Y, Tsuchida K, Shigemoto R, Nakanishi S (1991) Sequence and expression of a metabotropic glutamate receptor. Nature 349:760-765. ISSN 0028-0836

Matsuda LA, Bonner TI, Lolait SJ (1993) Localization of cannabinoid receptor mRNA in rat brain. Journal of Comparative Neurology 327:535-550. ISSN 1096-9861

Meldrum, B.S. (2000). Glutamate as a neurotransmitter in the brain: review of physiology and pathology. Journal of Nutrition 130:1007S-1015S. ISSN: 0022-3166

Nickell, W.T., Behbehani, M.M., and Shipley, M.T. (1994). Evidence for GABAB-mediated inhibition of transmission from the olfactory nerve to mitral cells in the rat olfactory bulb. Brain Research Bulletin 35:119-123. ISSN 0361-9230

Nicoll R, Alger BE (2004) The brain's own marijuana. Scientific American 291:68-75

Ohno-Shosaku T, Maejima T, Kano M (2001) Endogenous cannabinoids mediate retrograde signals from depolarized postsynaptic neurons to presynaptic terminals. Neuron 29:729-738. ISSN 0896-6273

Ohno-Shosaku T, Shosaku J, Tsubokawa H, Kano M (2002) Cooperative eCB production by neuronal depolarization and group I metabotropic glutamate receptor activation. European Journal of Neuroscience 15:953-961. ISSN 0953-816X

Ohno-Shosaku T, Matsui M, Fukudome Y, Shosaku J, Tsubokawa H, Taketo MM, Manabe T, Kano M (2003) Postsynaptic M1 and M3 receptors are responsible for the muscarinic enhancement of retrograde endocannabinoid signalling in the hippocampus. European Journal of Neuroscience 18:109-116. ISSN 0953-816X

Ohishi H, Shigemoto R, Nakanishi S, Mizuno N (1993) Distribution of the mRNA for a metabotropic glutamate receptor, mGluR2, in the central nervous system of the rat. Neuroscience 53:1009-1018. ISSN 0306-4522

Ohishi H, Neki A, Mizuno N (1998) Distribution of a metabotropic glutamate receptor, mGluR2, in the central nervous system of the rat and mouse: an immunohistochemical study with a monoclonal antibody. Neuroscience Research 30:65-82. ISSN 0168-0102

Ohishi H, Akazawa C, Shigemoto R, Nakanishi S, Mizuno N (1995) Distributions of the mRNAs for L-2-amino-4-phosphobutyrate-sensitive metabotropic glutamate receptors, mGluR4 and mGluR7, in the rat brain. Journal of Comparative Neurology 360:555-570. ISSN 1096-9861

Panikashvili D, Simeonidou C, Ben-Shabat S, Hanus L, Breuer A, Mechoulam R, Shohami E (2001) An endogenous cannabinoid (2-AG) is neuroprotective after brain injury. Nature 413:527-531. ISSN 0028-0836

Petralia, R.S., Wang, Y.X., Singh, S., Wu, C., Shi, L., Wei, J., and Wenthold, R.J. (1997). A monoclonal antibody shows discrete cellular and subcellular localizations of mGluR1 alpha metabotropic glutamate receptors. Journal of Chemical Neuroanatomy 13:77-93. ISSN: 0891-0618

Pistis M, Perra S, Pillolla G, Melis M, Gessa GL, Muntoni AL (2004) Cannabinoids modulate neuronal firing in the rat basolateral amygdala: evidence for CB1- and non-CB1-mediated actions. Neuropharmacology 46:115-25. ISSN 0028-3908

Puche AC, Shipley MT (2001) Radial glia development in the mouse olfactory bulb. Journal of Comparative Neurology 434:1–12. ISSN 1096-9861

Romano C, Sesma MA, McDonald CT, O'Malley K, van den Pol AN, Olney JW (1995) Distribution of metabotropic glutamate receptor mGluR5 immunoreactivity in rat brain. Journal of Comparative Neurology 355:455-469. ISSN 1096-9861

Sahara Y, Kubota T, Ichikawa M (2001) Cellular localization of metabotropic glutamate receptors mGluR1, 2/3, 5 and 7 in the main and accessory olfactory bulb of the rat. Neuroscience Letters 312:59-62. ISSN 0304-3940

Salt, T.E., Turner, J.P., and Kingston, A.E. (1999). Evaluation of agonists and antagonists acting at group I metabotropic glutamate receptors in the thalamus in vivo. Neuropharmacology 38:1505-1510. ISSN 0028-3908

Saugstad JA, Kinzie JM, Shinohara MM, Segerson TP, Westbrook GL (1997) Cloning and expression of rat metabotropic glutamate receptor 8 reveals a distinct pharmacological profile. Molecular Pharmacology 51:119-125. ISSN 0026-895X

Schoepp, D.D., and Conn, P.J. (1993). Metabotropic glutamate receptors in brain function and pathology. Trends in Pharmacological Sciences 14:13-20. ISSN 0165 -6147

Schoppa NE, Westbrook GL (1999) Regulation of synaptic timing in the olfactory bulb by an A-type potassium current. Nature Neuroscience 2:1106-1113. ISSN 1097-6256

Schoppa NE, Kinzie JM, Sahara Y, Segerson TP, Westbrook GL (1998) Dendrodritic inhibition in the olfactory bulb is driven by NMDA receptors. Journal of Neuroscience 18:6790-6802. ISSN 0270-6474

Shepherd GM, Chen WR, Greer CA (2004) Olfactory bulb. In: The synaptic organization of the brain, 5th ed, GM Shepherd ed, Oxford University Press, New York, pp 165-216. ISBN 0-19-515956-X

Shigemoto R, Nakanishi S, Mizuno N (1992) Distribution of the mRNA for a metabotropic glutamate receptor (mGluR1) in the central nervous system: an in situ hybridization study in adult and developing rat. Journal of Comparative Neurology 322:121-135. ISSN 1096-9861

Shipley MT, Ennis M (1996) Functional organization of olfactory system. Journal of Neurobiology 30:123-176. ISSN 0022-3034

Stella N, Schweitzer P, Piomelli D (1997) A second endogenous cannabinoid that modulates long-term potentiation. Nature 388:773-778. ISSN 1097-6256

Takahashi KA, Linden DJ (2000) Cannabinoid receptor modulation of synapses received by cerebellar Purkinje cells. Journal of Neurophysiology 83:1167-1180. ISSN 0022-3077

Thompson SM, Kao JP, Kramer RH, Poskanzer KE, Silver RA, Digregorio D, Wang SS (2005) Flashy science: controlling neural function with light. Journal of Neuroscience 25:10358-65. ISSN 0270-6474

Trettel J, Levine ES (2003) Endocannabinoids mediate rapid retrograde signaling at interneuron right-arrow pyramidal neuron synapses of the neocortex. Journal of Neurophysiology 89:2334-2338. ISSN 0022-3077

Trettel J, Fortin DA, Levine ES (2004) Endocannabinoid signalling selectively targets perisomatic inhibitory inputs to pyramidal neurones in juvenile mouse neocortex. Journal of Physiology (London) 556:95-107. ISSN 0022-3751

Tsou K, Mackie K, Sanudo-Pena MC, Walker JM (1999) Cannabinoid CB1 receptors are localized primarily on cholecystokinin-containing GABAergic interneurons in the rat hippocampal formation. Neuroscience 93:969-975. ISSN 0306-4522

Valjent E, Mitchell JM, Besson MJ, Caboche J, Maldonado R (2002) Behavioural and biochemical evidence for interactions between Delta9-tetrahydrocannabinol and nicotine. British Journal of Pharmacology 135:564-578. ISSN 0007-1188

van den Pol A (1995) Presynaptic metabotropic glutamate receptors in adult and developing neurons: autoexcitation in the olfactory bulb. Journal of Comparative Neurology 253-271. ISSN 1096-9861

Varma N, Carlson GC, Ledent C, Alger BE (2001) Metabotropic glutamate receptors drive the endocannabinoid system in hippocampus. Journal of Neuroscience 21:(RC188) 1-5. ISSN 0270-6474

Wada E, Shigemoto R, Kinoshita A, Ohishi H, Mizuno N (1998) Metabotropic glutamate receptor subtypes in axon terminals of projection fibers from the main and accessory olfactory bulbs: a light and electron microscopic immunohistochemical study in the rat. Journal of Comparative Neurology 393:493-504. ISSN 1096-9861

Wilson RI, Nicoll RA (2001) Endogenous cannabinoids mediate retrograde signalling at hippocampal synapses. Nature 410:588-592. ISSN 0028-0836

Wilson RI, Kunos G, Nicoll RA (2001) Presynaptic specificity of endocannabinoid signaling in the hippocampus. Neuron 31:1-20. ISSN 0896-6273

Yoshida T, Hashimoto K, Zimmer A, Maejima T, Araishi K, Kano M (2002) The cannabinoid CB1 receptor mediates retrograde signals for depolarization-induced suppression of inhibition in cerebellar Purkinje cells. Journal of Neuroscience 22:1690-1697. ISSN 0270-6474

Zhu PY, Lovinger DM (2005) Retrograde endocannabinoid signaling in a postsynaptic neuron/synaptic bouton preparation from basolateral amygdala. Journal of Neuroscience 25:6199-6207. ISSN 0270-6474

Section 2

Cognitive and Social Neuroscience

3

Neuropsychological Context of Marital Functioning

Jan Rostowski[1] and Teresa Rostowska[2]
[1]High School of Finance and Management, Faculty of Psychology in Warsaw
[2]University of Gdansk, Institute of Psychology
Poland

1. Introduction

Current achievements in neuroscience prove that when it comes to human behavior, human brain is responsible for solving social problems by activating psychological executory mechanisms aimed at specific problems, which developed thanks to the processes of natural selection. This kind of approach assumes modularity of brain's functioning. The modular approach posits that brain comprises of modules of different and diverse neuronal centers and processes and mechanisms for solving different social problems connected to them. And so for example learning processes or different forms of cognition work accordingly to different principles or rules, by using different complex neuronal structures and programs to process information; for example, different ones about words, others about faces or another ones about smells, and about sounds, etc. In that way a modular approach understood assumes that people can notice, remember and evaluate information in different ways and also decide on different ways of using it to carry out different social goals (Sundie et al., 2006). This particular propriety has an important meaning for explaining and understanding complex social processes in general, and in particular, for functioning of an intimate relationship, for example a marriage. This is why the issues concerning marriage and family should be also examined in a multisystem context of the life of its members. However, in practice and in a traditional approach, researching and investigating this phenomenon is limited to socio-cultural macro-systems in which those institutions function. What is usually not taken into consideration is the micro-system level of analysis that includes internal experience of the partners or family members seen as a class of brain processes. Thanks to dynamic advancements of research techniques, the scope of neuropsychological knowledge widened significantly in the last years, enabling a better and broader understanding of human brain functioning and its influence on all the forms or signs of human psyche and behavior that take place in close interpersonal relationships, and more particularly in marriages. It is thus not surprising that some researchers propose to describe it as 'interpersonal neurobiology', consequently underlining the meaning of relation between the interpersonal relationships, emotions and the brain. Understanding the key concepts of social neuropsychology can significantly enrich the work of psychologists on the problems of married couples or families both in theoretical, as well as in practical aspects, and mostly in the therapeutic aspect and even clinical one (Fishbane, 2007; Atkinson, 2005).

Human brain that is equipped with millions of neurons, connected with each other with billions of chemical synapses, is the most complex unit in the Universe. What is more important, those connections create neuronal circuits, that form neuronal networks in different parts of the brain. Activation of those circuits in specific, but different areas of the brain, causes an appearance of specific but diverse processes of thought, emotion and action, since, as it turns out, brain functions in a modular way. It must be noted that experiences which originated in interaction with the environment, influence the development of the brain through changes or through creating new connections in already existing neuronal circuits during the whole lifespan of an individual, thanks to the neuroplasticity that is characteristic for the human brain. Especially early experiences coming from the relation parent - child can indirectly modify the activity of genes responsible for the development and forming of particular brain structures. This process is crucial for shaping of different forms of attachment. It should be noted that already shaped brain structures, i.e. neuronal circuits and neuronal networks that influence or even determine preferences, personality and strategies for acting and for keeping oneself alive, were activated and included in circuits early on and are not very prone to or are even resistant to change, as they are the neuronal basis of habits, that allow for relatively permanent and predictable forms of actions and behaviors (Ito et al., 2007; Cunningham , Johnson, 2007; Goleman, 2006).

In close interpersonal relationships, especially marital ones, the key role is of the emotions-feelings-affects. It should be also noted, that neuronal structures responsible for human emotions are not localized in one, singular area of the brain, but contained in numerous interconnected circuits . The majority of the information on the emotional sphere is processed unconsciously and subcortially, mainly in the limbic system. Usually one is not aware of the fact that emotional processes take place during real-time in one's brain; only after they reach the level of cortex one becomes aware of them and they are properly interpreted as specific pieces of data originating in structures of the limbic system and in other brain structures, or even in other structures of the rest of the body. Because of that, in terms of neuroscience there is a distinction between emotions and feeling and affects. Emotions, being an evolutional adaptation, are unconscious and are linked to somatic processes, i.e. somatic expressions typical for each of the emotions - mostly facial expression and body posture; as stated by LeDoux (1995) emotions 'are full of blood, sweat and tears' and mostly happen on a subcortical level. It is worth mentioning that the commonly found emotions are: love-concern, joy-happiness, sadness, fear, disgust, surprise, anger. While feelings have a character or a form of emotions' content, however, what is important, are processes on a cortical and conscious level without the accompanying somatic processes. Humans have a limited ability to define their feelings; so far around 35 feelings were named. A neurological case of lack of the ability to identify or utter the emotional content in a form of feelings is known as alexithymia. While the affects have a processed, mostly on the level of prefrontal cortex of the frontal lobe, content form of feelings connected with a system of values and aims and with a clear influence on behavior and actions of an individual, affects also lasts longer; they are one of the executive functions of the prefrontal cortex. When examining the course of processes of emotional stimuli of the emotions-feeling sphere, what must be taken into consideration is the so called bottom way on the level of subcortical structures and after that a transmission to the cerebral cortex, i.e. 'bottom-up' and an upper way on the level of the cerebral cortex and transmission of the information to the subcortical structures, i.e. 'top-down' (see: Rostowski, 2007). What is very important for the parameters of interpersonal relationships is not only the capacity but also the ability to adequately communicate to each other the positive feelings. However, in this respect, there are individual differences partially determined by inherited-genetic factors, as for example in the case of introverts and extraverts (Morris, Cacioppo, 2007; Fishbane, 2007; Liebermann, 2007; Ochsner, 2007).

As aforementioned, social neuropsychology, in a detailed way, includes forms of social behaviors of individuals, although with a close relationship or a strong reference to functioning of particular brain structures, i.e., specific neuronal circuits. Within a framework outlined above, what will be considered in this part are some of the more important forms of behaviors in married life and their possible influences on the functioning quality of marriages or other interpersonal relationships. The forms of social behaviors studied here, can be different depending on whether the particular brain structures were formed properly or improperly, whether they were shaped in a disturbed way and with deficits and, which defines or determines the expressions or forms of behavior as either correct, socially acceptable and expected or incorrect, poor, visibly disturbed and pathologic, influencing the quality of functioning of partners in a marriage or in other interpersonal relationships.

Using this approach, in this chapter, the following processes will be examined: self-control, imitation (simulation), empathy, self-knowledge, mind reading (mentalization) and the role of mirror neurons in perceiving oneself and other people - as the direction of their development and the levels of their intensity decide, to a big extent, on the character of the relation between the partners of interaction and thus on the quality of functioning of a marriage.

2. Self-regulation

A very important human ability in civilized societies, and even more so in institutions or social groups, and especially in close interpersonal relationships, like marriage, that are characterized by a need of constant interaction between the partners - is the ability to regulate and control one's thoughts, feelings or actions. This approach considers self-regulation as higher level executive control, i.e. concerning executory functions like: predicting, planning, setting goals, restraining or consciously planning actions, executing, concentrating, working memory, making choices or decisions, naturally, in relation to lower, first level processes, i.e. subcortical processes. That being said, self-regulation mostly relates to control of emotions, feelings, instincts, needs, impulses or motivations. Admittedly, people have the ability to delay gratification and to control their inclinations-desires and to pursue goals; yet it is the failure of self-regulation in everyday life, usually intoxicant abuse-drunkenness, gluttony, different forms and different degrees of domestic violence, arguments, conflicts, etc, that is the most important and the most frequent cause of the troubles concerning marriage, family and society. It should be noted that self-regulation is also very important for all aspects of mental and physical health, and also disorders in those areas. This is why understanding the nature of self-regulation, both in the aspect of its successful implementation, as well as on the failure side, can bring valid insight into the conditions for its positive course, execution and for its failure and the potential to prevent failure from happening (Cacioppo et al., 2007; Decety, 2007; Engelberg & Sjoberg, 2005; Rostowski, 2008).

The results of social-cognitive neuropsychology studies enrich the knowledge and the understanding of neuronal mechanisms of self-regulation. It turns out that they cover three basic prefrontal neuronal circuits that are related to executive functions, that is: 1 ventromedial/ orbitofrontal prefrontal cortex, 2 dorsolateral prefrontal cortex and 3. anterior cingulate cortex. A number of processes depend on those three neuronal circuits, and especially on the anterior cingulate cortex, namely the processes connected with self-regulation of behaviors important in interpersonal relations, especially in marriages, like: monitoring the process of decision making, initiating the choice of new, but correct reaction from numerous alternatives, monitoring activities and the results of execution, detecting and generating adequate reactions in conflict situations, predicting the possibilities of making mistakes, estimating the benefits or rewards and losses or punishments, or perceiving physical, social and psychological suffering, so actions that have the key meaning in marriage and family life. Damaging the aforementioned neuronal structures or lowering their level of functional activation, causes deterioration of related self-regulation and restraining processes, that is, the processes of restrain during the interaction between the partners. And cases of severe damages can cause serious mental disorders like depression or personality disorders, mood disorders, decrease in self-awareness, emotional instability, apathy and other serious disruptions of social behaviors. That is, behaviors that affect the course and climate of everyday life, not to mention its quality. In extreme cases it can cause obsessive-compulsive disorder or even schizophrenia (Cacioppo et al., 2007; Ochsner, 2007; Decety, 2007).

3. Self-re-evaluation

When it comes to close interpersonal relationships, especially marriages, what matters greatly for correct social functioning in them is self-regulation of emotions, and especially self-regulation of negative emotions. It is worth mentioning that currently, cognitive approach perceives emotions' self-regulation as reappraisal (according to Lazarus - secondary appraisal) that lies in reinterpretation of meaning of the same emotional incident, although in non-emotional categories, but basing it on the processes on awareness level. It should be noted that using this secondary appraisal of events of an emotional-sentimental nature, can have an important impact on shaping correct or incorrect interpersonal relations within the married couple, or between the members of other social groups. The core of this process is in a way a cognitive transformation/ a change of negative emotions induced on a subcortical level with unpleasant events by reexamining them again on a cerebral cortex level in other, more objective categories of actual state, due to which they loose their primary, aversive-unpleasant character or dimension, and at the same time, an individual looses those unpleasant emotions, for example fear, anger, sadness, jealousy, etc. Neuronal structures responsible for this process of secondary appraisal of aversive stimuli is 1.lateral prefrontal cortex and 2.different areas of medial prefrontal cortex and 3. anterior cingulate cortex as well as 4. dorsomedial prefrontal cortex, that all together participate in - on one hand - cognitive control processes, and on the other - they deactivate, by restraining structures responsible for inducing negative emotional reactions, for example anxiety or depression on a subcortical level. For those sometimes negative reactions the mainly responsible structures are: 1.amygdala, 2.partially hippocampus and 3. orbitomedial prefrontal cortex. It turns out that the above-mentioned medial prefrontal cortex is basically responsible for shaping the strategy of secondary appraisal through modulating the activity of different systems connected to processing or examining emotional states (Cacioppo et al., 2007; Decety, 2007; Ochsner, 2007; Ochsner et al., 2002).

In order to get to know and understand better the course of those two-level process-reactions when examining the role of subcortical and cerebral cortex role in emotion processing, two ways of emotional activity have to be taken into consideration that are also connected to the process of emotional self-regulation. According to the concept suggested by LeDoux (2000, 1995), that is the bottom -up way, which is a quick, unaware system, of a reactive character of processing emotional information. Thanks to that quick processing there is an 'instinctive' evaluation, basically on a limbic system level, and, to be exact, on an amygdala level, of possibility of threat, or a specific danger and activate reactions that protect individual from possible harm.. This quick protective reaction happens, among other things, through appearance of bio- or somatic markers in a form of a sometimes vague feeling, consequences, outcomes of a situation, event – in a physiologic-somatic sphere, for example sweating (that is a psychogalvanic reflex). It is mostly a way from amygdala to cerebral cortex, and so the way 'bottom-up'. However there also is an 'upper-better-main way' that is 'top-down', which means from the level of cerebral cortex structures, mostly prefrontal ones, to subcortical structures, mainly to amygdala; that lies in reaction to emotional stimuli that is reflexive, cautious, thought through and with a certain delay after which decisions are made which are more consistent with the situation (Ochsner, 2007; Atkinson, 2005; Rostowski, 2008).

Cerebral cortex structures that mostly take part in this process of 'upper way' and to be more exact in the process of emotions regulation are functions connected to 1. ventromedial prefrontal cortex and 2. orbitoprefrontal cortex. Ventromedial prefrontal cortex, together with bilateral connections with other brain areas, plays a key part in the processes of emotional-affective regulation and self-regulation. In the light of the research, it turns out that people with damages to this structure of prefrontal cortex often make social errors, take tactless actions and commit faux pas in their interpersonal actions and behaviors, due to lack of control over their own emotions and lack of recognition of other people's emotions, lack of empathy, intuition or attention, as well due to apathy, emotional instability, and lack of adjustment of autonomic functions (Decety, 2007; Lieberman, 2007). While, when it comes to orbitofrontal prefrontal cortex, what should be noted is the process of affecting amygdala in a calming and restraining way, which allows for making decisions by choosing an alternative, and as a consequence, decisions compliant or subordinated to values' system and aims, and in a broader sense to correct action strategy of an individual in interpersonal relations. In light of conducted studies, it turns out that orbitofrontal cortex can support manifestations of appropriate and correct forms of social behavior through numerous and different forms of constant monitoring of this behavior, especially in its relation to and its compatibility with social norms, as well as limiting the degree to which emotions influence cognitive processes. Cases of damage to the orbitofrontal cortex (not only structural but also functional, for example in a form of decreased demand for oxygen hypoxia, that is the so called 'Cool down' (BOLD)) can cause weakening and a reduction of this process of monitoring and insight into oneself. Thus damage to the orbitofrontal cortex limits the possibility of inducing the so called social emotions, e.g., those of shame, uneasiness or the feeling of committing a tactless action, and others, that is emotions crucial for motivating the process of making corrections of those socially incorrect, unsuitable, improper forms of behaviors in interpersonal relationships. And so, for example, people with damages to orbitofrontal cortex, in the context of spontaneous social interactions, display a tendency not only to act improperly but also to induce incorrect emotions. The emotions strengthen rather than correct the inaccurate social behaviors. For example, in the cases of displaying forms of behaviors objectively socially unsuitable, like, among others, teasing, irritating or making fun of others, excessive criticism, humiliating and putting down others, those people as a result of this type of improper behavior, do not feel uncomfortable, but more proud of this kind of behavior, this kind of semi showing off, rather characteristic for psychopathic behaviors. Unfortunately, these types of behaviors are sometimes present in marital conflicts (Beer, 2007; Beer et al., 2006; Fishbane, 2007; Ochsner, 2007).

It turns out, that the bottom way, i.e., the way from the limbic system, allows people for a fast, instinctive evaluation of threat and protects from it, often through impulsive reactions. While, according to LeDoux, the 'upper way' from the cerebral cortex level, allows for evaluation that is less reflexive, more thought through and more connected to choice. But a fast, usually unaware or subconscious evaluation of the situation, with the involvement of amygdala, is in fact unaware, but a 'highly adaptive reaction' that holds a significant meaning for keeping one alive and for an individual's functioning, by warning him or her in time of the impending danger. The integrated combined activity of the limbic system with prefrontal cortex, especially with the ventromedial prefrontal cortex, assures emotional and relational well-being.The integrated link with orbitofrontal prefrontal cortex allows for making choices in accordance with the aims and values displayed by an individual. It has to be added, that this part of the cerebral cortex has a significant meaning in the process of self-awareness, empathy, prediction (mental vision). What is more, this part of cerebral cortex is characterized by neuroplasticity, and its development occurs during the whole life-span through keeping the ability for changes on a neuronal level. It is worth mentioning, that this kind of development change occurring at an advanced age, seems to be the basis for existence of crystallized intelligence according to R. Cattell (1963, 1971) and especially the so called 'wisdom of old age'. On the other hand, traumatic experience in the early stages of an individual's life, mistreatment, sexual abuse, exploitation or neglect can diminish the functioning of orbitoprefrontal cortex or weaken its control influence on the amygdala. Especially in this kind of cases, and even when the prefrontal cortex is developed correctly, the influence of amygdala can take over the prefrontal cortex, like in the cases of sudden overflow of emotions, so called anger furies, aggression, and can overpower conscious thinking, weakening significantly or, in extreme cases eliminating, conscious control over emotions and resulting in negative outcomes, as it sometimes happens in the case of fury – anger or aggression fit, that can also happen in close partnerships and family relationships. This is mainly the result of neuronal connections of the amygdala with prefrontal cortex (and so 'bottom - up') that are more developed than the connections from prefrontal cortex to the amygdala (so 'top - bottom'). The opposite is the case for over-activity of the orbito-prefrontal cortex when blocking of a behavior happens, a kind of 'anchoring' of behavior of an individual on one way of acting, with a visible emotional component. This kind of cases is found in obsessive-compulsive disorders (Cacioppo et al., 2007; Cacioppo & Berntson, 2005; Heberlein & Adolphs, 2007; Rostowski, 2008).

4. Simulation – Imitation

In interpersonal relations and even more so in close interpersonal relationships like marriage, the process that has a key meaning is the process of simulation, or to express it differently, the process of imitation. Imitation is a form of learning of the widest application in development, allowing for acquiring many skills without loosing time that would be needed when learning in a trial and error process. Even more important, imitation is of a core significance and plays a part in the development of basic social skills, like reading facial expressions and other body gestures, and most importantly, understanding of goals, intentions, desires and wishes of other people; overall, it plays a key part in terms of social cognition. Currently there are a number of approaches of a neuropsychological character that attempt to explain the process of imitation. In accordance with the main assumptions, recognition of the emotional expressions of another person depends, at least partially, on a type of a subsystem of the same neuronal structures that were engaged and took part in the process of the expression of this emotion. In other words, the process of recognition of somebody's emotional expression by an observer in a way includes imitation of the observed emotion in his or her own neuronal brain circuits, connected to or responsible for inducing emotions. In the process of imitation, there is a type of 'emphatic' resonance. This type of resonance can even occur on an unconscious or subliminal level (Heberlein & Adolphs, 2007, Turner, 2007: Havet-Thomassin et al., 2006). The significance of the imitation process comes from the existence of a very complex and diverse network of interactions that is generated by the social world, which challenges people. The chance to be up to the challenge depends on the abilities of members of a particular community to understand one another. This claim is even more up-to-date and important, because remaining in and succeeding in such complex relationships like marriages or other close interpersonal relationships, depends on the degree to which the partners can understand each other and read or anticipate each other's social intentions, needs and desires. It should be noted that in the last years, neuropsychology addresses this issue and gradually offers ideas for explanation of ways due to which social cognition and understanding of others is possible, taking into consideration a proper functioning of the brain. An important step was discovering mirror neurons systems, that are neuronal and cognitive mechanisms of content information transfer. It happens when the activation state of a particular neuronal network that is the basis for activity for one person, is shared at the same time by another person. This concept assumes that the systems of mirror neurons are the main mechanisms for imitation-simulation, and are one of the most important neuronal systems, thanks to which understanding or imitating other people is achieved on the level of structures of functions of the brain itself. It happens as a result of a kind of close connection and 'transmission' from one brain to the other brain (that of another person), or even with numerous other brains, affecting not only the brain but, through activation of particular cerebral structures, also the body, in terms not only of cognition but also of actions or behaviors, as it happens, for example, when somebody meets or encounters another person, especially a close one. Higher level of mirror neuron activation usually accompanies execution of a particular activity or behavior, not only its observation. What should be taken into consideration, are two levels of accordance between the observed and the executed action when it comes to the unit/pattern of activation of mirror neurons that is close one and widened one. In case of close compatibility, the set of activated neurons is almost identical in the process of execution, as well as observing or imitating activity; while in the case of widened compatibility, the set of activated mirror neurons is not necessary the same, but similar enough that it allows for reaching the same goal; for example, a behavior of a mother and a child when greeting each other (a mother and a child behave a bit differently, but they both end up hugging each other). In the light of the neurology research results, it turns out that people's mirror neurons together with the higher visual areas in the brain structure, including superior temporal sulcus, create basic cortex circuits for the imitation processes. In this way, 1.circuits of superior temporal sulcus provide or assure higher level visual description of activity that is to be imitated, while 2. inferior parietal cortex as a second component of mirror neurons is connected to motor aspects of imitated activity and 3. inferior frontal cortex (Broca's area) is the third component of mirror neurons that is connected to recognition and the aim of the imitated activity. Though those cerebral cortex structures are strongly connected anatomically and functionally, they are not enough to explain and understand all of the activities, especially those linked to implementation of the imitation process, and even less to explain the social cognition connected to activity of mirror neurons. The participation of prefrontal cortex structures is also necessary (Jacoboni & Dapretto, 2006; Jacoboni, 2007; Fishbane, 2007; Lizardo, 2007).

It should be explained, in order to avoid misunderstandings, that those systems of mirror neurons are not the only means thanks to which a full social understanding and cognition is reached; next to those systems, to reach more complete social understanding, a semantic system is used, based on reasoning, using memory content, previous experiences, co-occurring context, etc. It should be emphasized that those two systems do not exclude each other, but rather complement one another, they are functionally complementary within the activities and executive functions of prefrontal cortex of frontal lobe (Muthukumaraswany, Johnson, 2007; Fishbane, 2007: Turner 2007).

5. Empathy

Activity of the presented above mirror neurons plays an important role in social cognition and is closely, specifically but complementary, related to empathy process expressed in close interpersonal relationships. Role of mirror neurons also assumes a paradigm of observation and imitation of body expression as well as other forms of behavior. It is known, even based on daily observation that people tend to imitate others automatically when they participate in social interaction. This phenomenon is called 'chameleon effect' or parroting. However, research indicates that the more people tend to imitate the more they tend to empathize with others. Research indicates that one way to empathize is in a way self-incorporating the face expression and reactions and body postures of others. This happens due to functioning of mirror neurons. However, since empathy process also assumes the need of emotional processing of information-stimuli, turning on the limbic system, apart from mirror neurons, also plays major role. It is important because mirror neurons and limbic system - amygdala to be precise - are anatomically linked with cortex structure through insula. It can be assumed that basic neurological base of empathy - empathizing ability consists of: 1/. mirror neurons system, 2/.insula, 3/. amygdala. It needs to be said though that depending on what category of stimuli initiates the empathy process, other neuronal systems might be activated as well. In the model depiction (with regard to emotional area) processes related to empathy in terms of shared emotions consist of: 1/.

somatosensory, 2/. frontal-parietal, 3/.premotor and 4/.motor cortex where the mirror neuron activity is particularly present and also: 5/. limbic system and 6/. cerebellum. In contrast, in the mental states domain the important structures are: 1/. inferior parietal cortex, 2/. ventromedial - prefrontal cortex, 3/. dorsolateral prefrontal cortex, 4/. medial prefrontal cortex in frontal lobe, 5/. dorsal temporal sulcus and 6/. insular and frontal cingulate cortex, and also 7/. amygdala. (Decety, 2007; Carr et al., 2002; Shamay-Tsoory, 2007). Development of these structures and their functioning level determines greatly – though not exclusively – the ability to empathize with others, so-called re-introduction and internal imitating or simulating, that is simulating of actions perceived in others: actions, facial and body expressions as well as activities performed by other body parts equipped with effectors. It needs to be added though that according to research, activity of mirror neuron system can modify the activity of other structures in this system. They are also responsible for reflecting the sensory – motor aspects of empathy (Decety, 2007; Jacoboni & Dapretto, 2006; Jacoboni, 2007; Muthukumaraswany & Johnson, 2007).

More recent research indicates that the human system of mirror neurons codes information from a broader range of behaviors and activities than it was earlier assumed. It is not reduced to motor activity or simple simulation but involves secondary expression of emotions, pain and basic somatic sensation. Facial emotional expression - observed and registered - even though not perceived by an observer, is registered by electromyography; small spasms of relevant muscles take place. Those elusive and unperceived facial expressions appear even when an individual is not consciously aware that the stimulus is presented, either because of short exposition or usage of some masking form (e.g. because of reluctance or lack of focus). Sometimes, despite those obstacles or lack of direct observation, at least vague awareness of someone around experiencing certain emotions becomes present in the form of emotional atmosphere in a given moment or the phenomenon of 'emotional contagion'. The latter means that emotions are shared through activation of an emotional mirror neuron system, above others related to facial expression that induce similar emotions in an observer or observers. Therefore, when observed faces look sad, then the observers tend to describe themselves as sadder and the other way round: when the happy, joyous face is looked at, people tend to recognize themselves as happier. The magnitude of this effect depends on strength - intensity of emotions expressed on observed faces. This data suggests that mirror neuron systems for emotions are switched on automatically in observer rather than activated by cortical centers. Therefore, the process is not 'top-bottom' but 'bottom – up'; it can be said that we do not intend to be empathic but we become so in the given situational context. Moreover, current research conducted with brain neuroimaging techniques indicates the presence of some active, neuronal and mental simulating mechanism in the process of understanding emotional states in others (Beer, 2006; Shamay-Tsoory, 2007).

And thus for actor and observer's emotion of disgust/repulsion responsible is: 1/. insular cortex, for emotion of fear 2/. amygdala, for anger 3/. ventral striatum and basal ganglia, for observation and experience of pain 4/. anterior cingulate cortex and anterior insular cortex, for bodily somatosensory experience 5/. secondary somatosensory cortex in parietal lobe. Presence of such mechanism becomes even more significant when it is taken into account that cerebral neuronal circuits that are responsible for inducing given emotions are located in different brain areas. It turns out that the same insular cortex area that is activated through exposure to smells perceived by observers as disgusting is also activated by observation of repulsion, disgust expressed by others. It thus turns out that shared reconstruction of disgust takes place in insular cortex and is activated both when disgust is sensed by the actor and when it is observed by another person - an observer. Similar dependency is to be found in case of amygdala which is - as was already stated - activated when the fear is both experienced and observed in others. This fact accounts for shared representation of fear in amygdala both for an actor and an observer. In case of emotion of anger the significant neuronal basis is mostly ventral striatum and basal ganglia. The neuronal mechanism of mirror neurons functioning in the case of pain is more complicated. However, research indicates that anterior cingulate cortex and anterior insular cortex are active both when the pain is experienced and when the experience of pain is observed by other people, especially those who feel love towards the person in pain. Among those observers there are distinct reactions to be found that indicate the avoidance reactions that reflect or suggest the actor's attitude in the form of shudder or flinch with pain when seeing pain experienced by a close person. This indicates the fully empathic reaction of an observer towards an actor. In case of experiencing somatosensory sensations - e.g. touch - both in actor and an observer secondary somatosensory cortex is activated in parietal lobe, adequately to part of the body. Summing up the above data, it can be concluded that there are various systems of cerebral mirror neurons for a number of information fields that can be the subject of experience both for an actor and for an observer (Muthukumaraswany & Johnson, 2007; Fishbane, 2007; Decety, 2007; Jacoboni & Dapretto, 2006; Bucino et al., 2005).

6. Self-cognition – Self-reflection

Recent research indicates that the mirror neuron system also plays a key role in the self-perception or self-cognition process. This accounts for individual's self-concept creation and its impact on shaping interpersonal relationships with close ones or people in general. Similarly to the way that simulation of others' behavior is becoming possible due to existence of mirror neurons, also self-perception - that is perceiving one's own image, own diverse and multi-dimensional self - becomes possible. Therefore we can, in a way, see ourselves in the mirror of our mirror neuron system. This sometimes takes place during moments of deep self-reflection or contemplation-meditation and in consequence of those processes self-regulation becomes possible. Important circumstances when it comes to close interpersonal relationships - like marriage - are those when activation level of mirror neurons, in the above discussed areas, increases significantly when similarity between an actor and an observer exists. This usually takes place between spouses (especially when the level of functioning quality of relationship is high) or in groups, close relatives, friends and acquaintances. Sustaining positive cognition and self-belief can facilitate maintaining good mental condition, health, and enhance psychological immunology system which enables remaining free of negative life events and memories. Moreover, disorder of self-information processing accounts for the basis of many psychological disorders - especially depression - that often impact negatively on interpersonal interactions between partners. This results from, among others, negative functioning of cognitive filter, and specifically, certain neuronal structures. An important role is played here by prefrontal cortex that is responsible for subjective reactions to self and others and more generally to external surrounding reality and thus allows for effective operating in social environment. To be more specific, the key role is played by medial prefrontal cortex that is responsible for processing of self-information which means cognitive and emotional aspects of self-reflection. However, ventromedial anterior cingulate cortex is also responsible for the emotional sphere. Decrease in metabolism of this cortex and even more so, shrinkage of its capacity remains closely related to depression and other affective disorders and self-evaluation (Cacioppo et al., 2007; Jacoboni, 2007; Jacoboni & Dapretto, 2006; Gotlib et al., 2005).

7. Role of mirror neurons in perception of self and others

Theory of mind conception can be investigated in two significantly different ways. The first one is about cognitive schema of other person's physical being, based on available rather mentalizing observation of that person's behavior. In the second understanding - the one that is taken into account in this work - theory of mind refers to depicting mental states that are based on prediction and interpretation of behaviors of others through taking into account understanding of their different mind states, e.g., their beliefs, biases, attitudes, goals, desires or even images (Saxe & Konwisher 2002; Shamey-Tsoory, 2007, Frith, Frith, 2006).

In said context, mirror neuron systems also account for neuronal basis of theory of mind. According to the simulation theory and even more, the hypothesis of 'mirror-matching' systems that assumes key role of mirror neurons system in discussed here 'mind reading' process, it is assumed that people use their own mental mechanisms to predict or rather reflect, mental processes, emotional states or motor activities in others. Neuronal basis for these abilities is an activity of properly functioning structures of prefrontal cortex that consist of orbitoprefrontal cortex - more in right hemisphere - that is related to or responsible for process of inference about others based on understanding their mental and emotional states. Left hemisphere is more related to tendency to confabulation or rather over-interpretation, using incorrect definitions or divagating from actual state (from the topic). Also the role of medial prefrontal cortex is important; that cortex is responsible for drawing conclusions about mental states or behaviors of others, even those that refer to the past. However, this is only possible when left hemisphere is activated. This process plays significant role in functioning of interpersonal relationships because complex set of mutually related thoughts, feelings and behaviors is an important condition for creating and maintaining closeness in mutually satisfying relationships. It facilitates a few important processes: 1/. getting to know the partner through observing and listening to him/her; 2/. applying correct attribution, assuming or deducting based on mentalization that partner's actions are driven by concern and positive dispositions or intentions; 3/. acceptance, respect and reciprocity since both partners participate in the same process that takes place mutually-bilaterally continuously in time and not only on the conscious level but also subconscious one. It comes as no surprise then that high level of mentalization is a factor that leads to close and highly satisfying interpersonal relationships. Even if small distortions appear, the perception of relationship is related to higher satisfaction; or the inverse is true, but moderating variables are to be found. It turns out that partners in long-term relationships are more precise in reading minds and predicting higher relationship satisfaction than partners in short-term relationships. However, more precise mind reading is to be found among more egocentric individuals because it is related to lower satisfaction with close relationship and there is lower tendency to positive distortion of perception of its activity forms. According to research, partners in close marital relationships in 50% of times attach importance to precision of mutual evaluations of thoughts and feelings. Other relationships do not attach such great importance. However, the longer the length of marriage the lower the importance attached to precision of reading thoughts and feelings; this is due to the increased mutual trust and relying on one another as well as motivation to follow closely the discussion threads. Those discussions are more of social nature than strategic; the latter one is more characteristic for marital couples with shorter length of marriage. Moreover, there are individual differences in ability to read minds. Individuals with higher social intelligence as well as those with higher education level are more skilled in reading others' thoughts and feelings (Fletcher, 2002; Fletcher et al., 2006; Dindia & Emmers-Sommer, 2006; Jacoboni, 2007; Beer, 2006; Cacioppo, et al., 2007; Saxe & Konwisher 2005).

It needs to be added that hypothesis that applies to ability to read thoughts and feelings, and taking into consideration the mirror neuron system - or to be specific: mirror-matching - seems to be, up to the point, convergent with philosophical- phenomenological approach to intersubjectivity that is defined as shared understanding of happenings between individuals. As it turns out, intersubjectivity can be considered on different levels. On the neuro-psychological level, intersubjectivity between people is generated in every individual through series of mirror matching neuronal circuits. On the phenomenological-experimental level, intersubjectivity creates the feeling of similarity or empathy with others in society. Disorders in such defined intersubjectivity may lead to psychopathological disorders, like schizophrenia, autism, psychotism.

However, it needs to be strongly emphasized that in positive understanding, mirror neurons - or, in other words, neuronal mirror matching - indicate the existence of general feature or ability of human brain to renewed usage of neuronal information processing for similar purposes. This ability is to be found not only at the basis of imitating empathy but also imagination - and so visual, auditory and kinesthetic imagination - and, what is more important, even volitional processes and states. On the other hand though, possibilities related to mirror neurons may also - in the context of social cognition - account for a basis for distortions, using incorrect attributions, heuristics, biases, conflicts etc. Therefore, in the social cognition, it is necessary to use the systems of semantic analysis of social situations, taking into account not only temporal lobes, parietal lobes, temporal-parietal junction but most of all prefrontal cortex of frontal lobes and specifically prefrontal ventromedial cortex responsible mostly for correct processes of control and decision (Lizardo, 2007; Turner 2007; Muthukumaraswamy & Johnson, 2007; Saxe & Konwisher 2002).

8. Cerebral hemispheres' asymmetry

Neurological research conducted for more than 20 years, provides proofs that left and right cerebral hemispheres are specialized in execution of slightly different, but at the same time, mostly complementary tasks and have control over various psychological functions. In particular, researchers concentrate on asymmetry of frontal lobes functioning in both hemispheres. Research indicates that left hemisphere is relatively more active than right hemisphere when an individual experiences positive emotions, encounters pleasant, joyful events. On the contrary, right frontal lobe is more active when an individual experiences negative emotions and encounters unpleasant events. It needs to be added that this asymmetric tendency, present since early childhood, is stable and coherent in time and needs to be considered in terms of individual differences as a trait. It also indicates its genetic, biological basis. From a practical point of view, an individual that displays activity pattern typical for right frontal hemisphere may have lower threshold of reaction to negative emotions. In other words, said individual is more sensitive and susceptible to have the negative emotions induced when unpleasant events are encountered. Therefore, an even hardly emotionally significant event may induce negative feelings that incline an individual with dominant frontal cortex of right hemisphere to withdraw or avoid. These individuals are more susceptible to experience negative emotions such as breakdown, anxiety, sadness. An individual with activity pattern typical for frontal cortex of left hemisphere has, on the other hand, lower threshold of reaction and experience to positive emotions when pleasant events are encountered. In such an individual, even emotionally weak stimuli may induce and maintain positive, pleasant feelings like happiness, joy, enthusiasm. Those feelings incline such an individual to approach or take appropriate actions. Individuals with dominant right hemisphere are more prone to depression, to react negatively to unknown and new stimuli and situations but very positively to known and familiar stimuli. An opposite susceptibility - i.e. to experience positive emotions – is to be found among individuals with relative domination of left hemisphere frontal cortex. It needs to be clearly emphasized that relative domination of frontal lobe may determine certain action style, behavior or level of experienced content and happiness and most of all, dominant mood. There is no need to justify how significant and of what impact is the relative compatibility of frontal cortex domination of one hemisphere on the level of marital relationship functioning (Larsen & Buss, 2002; Harmon-Jones, 2007; Kalin et al, 2002).

9. Summary

The approach proposed in this paper – based on social neuroscience – does not confine the relevance of analyzing marriage and family functioning in the socio-cultural context but it aims at indicating those aspects that were so far often omitted or considered less important.

Analyses presented above indicate that considering cognitive, emotional and social behaviors of individuals that function in interpersonal relationships, including marriages and families, requires taking neuropsychological approach into account. Today, there is no doubt that structural and functional maturity of many cerebral structures and related to them neuronal circuits, determines functioning efficiency of basic cognitive processes - most of all perception, attention, memory, thinking, imagination - and also various subcortical and cortical structures that are mostly responsible for different emotional states. Newest achievements in modular cerebral functionality allow for explaining the role and significance of various neuropsychological processes and mechanisms that account for the basis of specific behaviors among spouses or family members, such as: self-regulation, empathy, self-cognition, mind reading and mentalization. All those processes account for fundamental basis of cognitive, emotional and social human behaviors and affect perception of self and others and thus nature, specific character and quality of interpersonal relationships that an individual experiences in own marital and family life.

10. References

Atkinson,B.,J., (2006), Emotional Intelligence in Couples Therapy. Advances from Neurobiology and the Science of Intimate Relationsips. New York, London. W.W. Norton & Company.

Beer, J. (2007). The Importance of Emotion-Social Cognition Interactions for Social Functioning: Insights from Orbitofrontal Cortex. In: E. Harmon-Jones, P. Winkielman (Eds). Social Neuroscience, pp. 15-30. New York: The Guilford Press

Beer, J. (2006). Orbitofrontal Cortex and Social Regulation. In; J. Cacioppo, P. Visser, C. Pickett (Eds). Social Neuroscience. People Thinking about People, pp. 153-166.Cambridge, The MIT Press

Beer, J. John, O., Scabini,D. & Knight, R. (2006). Orbitofrontal Cortex and Social Behavior: Integrating Self-monitoring and Emotion-Cognition Interactions. *Journal of Cognitive Neuroscience,*18, 871-879

Buccino, G., Binkofski, F., Fink, G., Fadiga, L., Fogassi, L.,Gallese, V., Seltz.,Zilles, K.,Rizzolatti, G. & Freund, H-J. (2005), Action Observation Activates Premotor and Parietal Areas in a Somatotopic Manner: An fMRI Study. In: J. Cacioppo, G. Berntson (Eds). Social Neuroscience, pp. 133-142. New York: Psychology Press

Cacioppo, J., Amaral, D., Blanchard, J. & et al., (18) (2007). Social Neuroscience. Progress and Implications for Mental Heath. *Perspectives on Psychological Science,* 2, 99-123

Cacioppo, J., & Berntson, G. (2005). Volume Overview: Analyses of the Social Brain through the Lens of Human Brain Imaging In: J. Cacioppo, G. Berntson (Eds). Social Neuroscience, pp. 1-17. New York: Psychology Press

Carr, L., Jaccoboni, M., Dubeau, M-C., Mazziotta, J., & Lenzi, G. (2002). Neural Mechanisms of Empathy in Humans: A Relay from Neural Systems for Imitation to Limbic Areas. In: J. Cacioppo, G. Berntson (Eds).Social Neuroscience, pp. 143-152. New York: Psychology Press

Cattell, R. (1971).Abilities: Their Structure, Growth and Action. Boston: Houghton-Mifflin

Cattell, R. (1963). Theory of fluid and crystallized Intelligence: Critical Experiment. *Journal of Educational Psychology,* 54, 1-22

Cunningham, W., & Johnson, M. (2007). Attitudes and Evaluation: Toward a Component Process Framework. In: E. Harmon-Jones, P. Winkielman (Eds). Social Neuroscience, pp. 227-245. NewYork: The Guilford Press

Decety, J. (2007). A Social Cognitive Neuroscience: Model of Human Empathy. In: E. Harmon-Jones, P. Winkielman (Eds). Social Neuroscience, pp. 246-270. New York: The Guilford Press

Dindia, K., & Emmers-Sommer. (2006). What Partners Do to Maintain Their Close Relationships. In: P. Noller, J. Feeney (eds). Close Relationships. Functions, Forms, and Processes, pp.305-325. New York:Psychology Press

Engelberg, E., & Sjoberg, L. (2005).Emotional Intelligence and Inter-Personal Skills. In: R. Schulze, R. Roberts Eds). Emotional Intelligence. An International Handbook, pp.289-307. Massachusetts: Hogrefe & Huber Publishers

Fishbane, D. (2007).Wired to Connect: Neuroscience, Relationships, and Therapy. *Family Process,* 46, 395-412

Fletcher, G, Simpson, J., & Boyes, A. (2006). Accuracy and Bias in Romantic Relationships: An Evolutionary and Social Psychological Analysis. In: M. Schaller, J. Simpson, &

D. Kenrick (Eds). Evolution and Social Psychology, pp. 189-210. New York: Psychology Press

Fletcher, G. (2002). The New Science of Intimate Relationships. Oxford: Blackwell Publishers Ltd

Goleman. D. (2006). Social Intelligence. The New Science of Human Relationships. New York: A Bantam Book

Gotlib, I., Sivers, H., Gabrieli, J., & Canli,T. (2005). Subgenual Anterior Cingulate Activation to Valenced Emotional Stimuli in major Depression. *NeuroReport,* 16, 1731-1734

Havet-Thomasin, V., Allain, P., Etcharry, F., & Le Gall, D. (2006).What about Theory of Mind after Severe Brain Injury. *Brain Injuty,* 20, 83-91

Herberlein, A., & Adolphs, R. (2007). Neurobiology of Emotion Recognition: Current Evidence for Shred Substrates. In: E. Harmon-Jones, P. Winkielman (Eds). Social Neuroscience, pp. 31-55. New York: The Guilford Press

Ito,T., Willadsen-Jensen, E., & Correll, J. (2007). Social Neuroscience and Social Perception. In: E. Harmon-Jones, P. Winkielman (Eds). Social Neuroscience, pp. 401-421. New York: The Guilford Press

Jacoboni, M. (2007). The Quiet Revolution of Existential Neuroscience. . In: E. Harmon-Jones, P. Winkielman (Eds). Social Neuroscience, pp. 439-453. New York: The Guilford Press

Jacoboni, M., & Dapretto, M. (2006). The Mirror System and the Consequences of its Dysfunction. *Nature Reviews. Neuroscience,* 7, 942-951

Kalin, N., Larson, C., Shelton, S., & Davidson, R. (2002). Asymmetric Frontal Brain Activity, Cortisol, and Behavior Associated with Fearful Temperament I Rhesus Monkeys. In: J. Cacioppo, G. Berntson (Eds). Foundations in Social Neuroscience, pp. 1039-1048. Cambridge: The MIT Press

Larsen, L., & Buss, D. (2002*). Personality Psychology. Domains of Knowledge about Human Nature*. Boston: McGraw-Hill

LeDoux, J. (2000). Emotion Circuits in the Brain. *Annual Reviews of Neuroscience,* 23, 155-184

LeDoux, J. (1995). Emotion: Clues from Brain *Annual Reviews of Psychology,* 46, 209-235

Lieberman, M. (2007). The X and C-Systems: The Neural Basis of Automatic and Controlled Social Cognition. In: E. Harmon-Jones, P. Winkielman (Eds). Social Neuroscience, pp. 290-315. New York: The Guilford Press

Lizardo, O. (2007). "Mirror Neurons", Collective Objects and the Problem of Transmission: Reconsidering Stephen Turner's Critique of Practice Theory. *Journal for the Theory of Social Behaviour.* 37, 319-350

Muthukumaraswamy, S , Johnson B. (2007) A Dual Mechanism Neural Framework for Social Understanding. Philosophcal Psychology. 20.43-63.

Norris, C., & Cacioppo, J. (2007). I know How You Feel: Social and Emotional Information Processing in the Brain. In: E. Harmon-Jones, P. Winkielman (Eds). Social Neuroscience, pp. 84-105. New York: The Guilford Press

Ochsner, K. (2007). How Thinking Controls Feeling: A Social Cognitive Neuroscience Approach. In: E. Harmon-Jones, P. Winkielman (Eds). Social Neuroscience, pp. 106-133. New York: The Guilford Press

Ochsner, K., Bunge, S., Gross, J., & Gabrieli, J. (2002). Rethinking Feelings: An fMRI Study on the Cognitive Regulation of Emotion. In: J. Cacioppo, G. Berntson (Eds). Social Neuroscience, pp. 133-142. New York: Psychology Press

Rostowski J. (2008), The Neuropsychological Basis of Social Inteligence . *Polish Journal of Social Science. 3 , 59-80.*

Rostowski J., (2007), The Selected Aspects of the Memory in a Neuropsychological Perspective. *Polish Journal of Social Science.* 2,. 63-98.

Saxe, R., & Kanwisher, N. (2002). People Thinking about Thinking People: The Role of the Temporo-Parietal Junction in "Theory of Mind". In: J. Cacioppo, G. Berntson (Eds). Social Neuroscience, pp. 171-182. New York: Psychology Press

Shamay-Tsoory, S. (2007). Impairent Empathy following Ventromedial Prefrontal Brain Damage. In: T. Farrow, P. Woodruff (Eds). Empathy in Mental Illness, p. 89-110. New York: Cambridge University Press.

Sundie, J., Cialdini, R., Griskevicius, V., & Kendrick, D. (2006). Evolutionary Social Influence. In: M. Schaller, J. Simpson, & D. Kenrick (Eds). Evolution and Social Psychology, pp. 287-316. New York: Psychology Press

Turner, S. (2007). Mirror Neurons and Practices: A Response to Lizardo. *Journal for the Theory of Social Behaviour,* 37, 351- 371

Section 3

Clinical and Cognitive Neuroscience

4

Apraxia: Clinical Types, Theoretical Models, and Evaluation

François Osiurak[1] and Didier Le Gall[2,3]
[1]*Laboratoire d'Etude des Mécanismes Cognitifs (EA 3082), Université Lumière Lyon 2,*
[2]*Laboratoire de Psychologie des Pays de la Loire (EA 4638), Université d'Angers,*
[3]*Unité de Neuropsychologie, Département de Neurologie, Centre Hospitalier Universitaire d'Angers, France*

1. Introduction

Apraxia is traditionally defined as a disorder of skilled movement that cannot be attributed to elementary sensorimotor deficit, aphasia or severe mental deterioration (De Renzi, 1989). This negative definition has led to integrate within the same framework a multitude of relatively different clinical manifestations, which have little in common with the kind of deficits to which it was originally applied (e.g., gaze apraxia, gait apraxia, trunk apraxia). These forms probably concern automatic movements and, therefore, will not be treated here. It is now largely admitted that some clinical signs are particularly useful for the diagnosis. First, the disorder affects the two sides of the body, even though the brain lesions are generally unilateral and more particularly located in the left (dominant) hemisphere. Second, the errors made by apraxics vary depending on the conditions of testing. For instance, apraxics can succeed in many circumstances, but fail when the movement must be executed to the clinician's request. In this frame, three categories of movement are regarded as relevant to the evaluation: Imitation of meaningless postures, pantomime production (i.e., demonstration of the use of a tool without the tool in hand) and actual tool use. Apraxia has been, and is still, subject to intense debate notably about its autonomy from elementary sensorimotor deficits and from higher-level cognitive processes. As a result, neurologists and neuropsychologists alike are commonly uncertain about the good way of assessing and interpreting it. In this chapter, we propose to address different issues relative to the notion of apraxia in light of recent developments made in the field.

The first part of the chapter will introduce two authors who made a significant, historical contribution to the notion of apraxia, namely Hugo Karl Liepmann and Norman Geschwind. Then, in the second part, we will present the cognitive models of apraxia that have emerged since 1980 (Buxbaum, 2001; Rothi, Ochipa, & Heilman, 1991; Roy & Square, 1985). Third, we will discuss recent data collected by Georg Goldenberg that raise a certain number of controversies about the cognitive models mentioned above (Goldenberg, 1995, 2003, 2009). In the sake of clarity, our discussion will deal with apraxic manifestations assessed only with tasks of imitation of meaningless gestures, pantomime production and actual tool use. Besides discussing the psychological bases of apraxia, lesion sites associated with the different forms or apraxia will also be treated all along the paper. We hope that this chapter will help clinicians and students to better understand what apraxia is and how to evaluate it.

2. Historical background

2.1 Liepmann (1908, 1920)

We owe the first description of apraxia to Jackson (1866), who observed a motor intentional deficit in aphasic patients. Those patients were unable to move the tongue or lips on command, but could carry out these movements in an automatic movement sequence such as swallowing or eating. Jackson observed that this automatic-voluntary dissociation was not restricted to muscles of the facial region, since some of those aphasic patients were also unable to move their right, non-plegic hand on command while the same actions could be performed correctly in a spontaneous way. Although the first observations of apraxic patients are credited to Jackson, it was Steinthal (1871; see also Gogol, 1873) who coined the term apraxia. He described the case of an aphasic patient who attempted to write by holding a pencil upside down, or manipulated a fork and a knife as if he had never used them before. Steinthal stressed that it was not the ability to perform movements of extremities which was defective, but rather the relationship between the movements and the manipulated object, thereby suggesting that the absence of action (i.e., "a-praxia") might result from a perceptual deficit affecting object use recognition.

These observations led authors to hypothesize that apraxia might be a single neurological syndrome to be distinguished from agnosia, aphasia or asymbolia. Nevertheless, clinical and experimental evidence was still not enough to support this hypothesis. In fact, many authors thought at that time that it was hard to differentiate between apraxia and elementary sensorimotor deficits such as paresis. Independence of apraxia from pure motor deficits was supported by the observation of a 48-year-imperial councillor, the patient MT, by Liepmann (1900). MT was aphasic and showed clear-cut apraxia of the right hand. The deficit affected the movements of right extremities as well as movements of the head, the face and the tongue. MT was however able to perform properly, with his left hand, gestures on verbal command and upon imitation, including tool use. Verbal comprehension, visual recognition and global intellectual functioning were largely preserved. Liepmann proposed the term "motor apraxia" to describe this particular impairment.

In 1908, Liepmann published a study including 42 right brain-damaged (RBD) patients and 47 left brain-damaged (LBD) patients. He found apraxia in 20 out of 47 LBD patients. He also stressed that it did not occur at all in the right hands of the group of RBD patients. Liepmann proposed to call "sympathetic apraxia" this kind of apraxia which accompanies right hemiplegia. Moreover, 14 out of 20 LBD patients with apraxia were aphasic, but 6 were not. So, he argued that the left cerebral hemisphere is dominant not only for language but also for motor control. He also suggested that apraxia often accompanies aphasia, but is independent of it. In the meanwhile, Pick (1905) reported the case of an aphasic patient who was able to understand simple instructions, name objects and explain their functional use, but could use a knife to comb his hair, put a match to the mouth in an attempt to smoke it or encounter severe difficulties to demonstrate how to use a key or a pair of scissors. Pick interpreted this disorder as a sign of motor apraxia given that the patient showed intact knowledge of functional uses of objects.

On the basis of these findings, Liepmann (1908, 1920) made the first clinical and anatomical synthesis of apraxia. He thought skilled movements to be supported by the creation of movement formulae in the whole posterior cortex. Movement formulae are constituted by acoustic or visual images of the action. To perform skilled movements, movement formulae produced by the posterior brain have to be associated via cortical connections with the innervatory patterns stored in the left sensorimotor region. When the left hand has to carry out the movement, the information is transferred via the corpus callosum to the right sensorimotor region. In sum, there is only one mechanism for skilled movements, which can nevertheless be impaired at three levels, thus producing three distinct forms of apraxia (Figure 1).

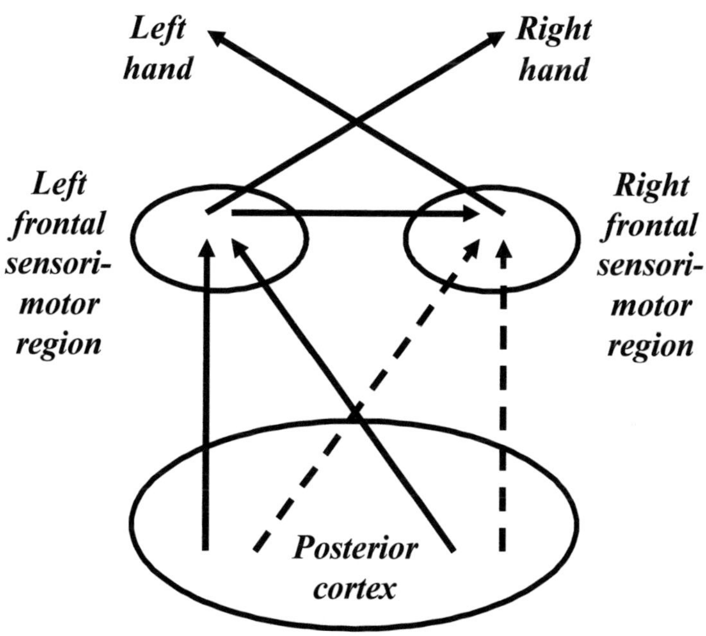

Fig. 1. First synthesis of Liepmann (1908) displaying the mechanism of apraxia. Explanations are given in the text. Adapted from Goldenberg (2009).

First, patients with "Ideational Apraxia" (IA or motor apraxia for Pick) fail to generate movement formulae and, therefore, show impairment in the real and pantomimed use of tools. Patients may however perform normally when provided with the idea of the gesture, such as when asked to carry out movements upon imitation. It was first thought to be a severe form of ideomotor apraxia (see below), but Liepmann confirmed its independence in 1920 and associated this disorder with lesions of the whole posterior cortex and, more particularly, the left posterior regions. Second, in "IdeoMotor Apraxia" (IMA or motor apraxia in the princeps study of 1900), movement formulae are intact but can no longer guide the innervatory patterns. In short, the patient knows what he has to do, but does not know how to do it. Patients with IMA show predominantly difficulties to perform meaningful gestures on verbal command and on imitation. Actual tool use is partly spared because of the adaptation of movements to external constraints. This form of apraxia was associated with the destruction of fibres connecting posterior brain regions to the frontal sensorimotor regions (callosal, frontal and parietal). Given that these fibres pass below the parietal cortex, Liepmann suggested that deep lesions of the inferior parietal lobe and the supramarginal gyrus may cause IMA (see Goldenberg, 2009). Third, "Motor Apraxia" (melo-kinetic apraxia in the paper of 1908) corresponds with the impairment of innervatory patterns. Contrary to IA and IAM that affect movements of both hands, motor apraxia is unilateral and occurs regardless of the conditions of evaluation (no automatic-voluntary dissociation). Motor apraxia is associated with lesions of frontal sensorimotor regions.

2.2 Geschwind (1965, 1975)

The disconnection approach was partly initiated by the description of the imperial counsellor MT by Liepmann (1900). The problem inherent to this description is that, unlike the patient MT, unilateral non-sympathetic apraxia affects more frequently the left upper limb than the right one. Geschwind (1965) developed his theoretical model of apraxia on this basis. Geschwind and Kaplan (1962) discussed the case of a patient with an extensive infarction of corpus callosum, who was able to write correctly with the right hand but not with the left hand, which did not show an elementary sensorimotor disturbance. Moreover, the patient could perform gestures on verbal command (pantomime) with the right hand but frequently failed to carry them out with the left hand. Importantly, he could imitate the movement made by the examiner as well as use objects correctly with either hand. The hypothesis that the failures of this patient resulted from a general conceptual disturbance was ruled out by the fact that the patient could pretend to use objects with the right hand. Instead, given that the difficulties occurred when the patient was asked to perform actions to command, Geschwind and Kaplan interpreted these disturbances as the effects of disconnection of the right motor cortex from the speech area and suggested that the extensive infarction of the corpus callosum must be regarded as the cause of the symptoms.

Geschwind (1965) stressed that this case did not represent the difficulties which usually accompany left unilateral apraxia. Indeed, impairment is generally not limited to gesture on verbal command and also occurs when patients are requested to imitate or to actually use tools. This is consistent with the first description of the clinical manifestation of extensive disconnection of the corpus callosum by Liepmann and Maas (1907). Their patient, Ochs, had a right hemiplegia. He could not write with his left hand and failed to perform many actions on verbal command and did not improve on imitation. Ochs also frequently mishandled objects placed in his left hand. So, Geschwind (1965, p. 606) emphasized that "the designation of "apraxic" is an inadequate one unless the stimulus conditions are specified...Rather than use the term "apraxia" it is therefore preferable to specify the stimulus-response combinations which fail".

A few years later, Geschwind (1975) proposed a neo-associationist model which diverted from Liepmann's theory in that he replaced the movement formulae by the verbal command which elicits motor actions by using a neural substrate similar to that used by Wernicke to language processing (Figure 2). Sensorial centres are directly linked to motor centres and apraxia is viewed as an interruption of the translation of sensorial stimulations into motor inputs. The Wernicke area is connected to the left motor association area by the arcuate fasciculus, and the left motor association area is linked to the left primary motor area. When a person is requested to perform a gesture on verbal command with the right hand, this pathway is used. If a person has to use the left hand, information is transferred from the left motor association area to the right motor association area and then to the right primary motor area. For Geschwind, lesions in the region of the arcuate fasciculus and supramarginal gyrus disconnect Wernicke area from motor association areas. So, patients with lesions in this area can comprehend verbal commands but show difficulties in carrying out movements to command with either hand. Gesture-to-command but not imitation requires left hemisphere language processing. So, given that many LBD patients have no right hemisphere lesion, they should be able to imitate, but cannot. To account for this discrepancy, Geschwind suggested that the left arcuate fasciculus is also dominant for visuomotor connections. Finally, callosal lesions produce a unilateral apraxia of the left hand, as described by Geschwind and Kaplan (1962) and Liepmann and Maas (1907).

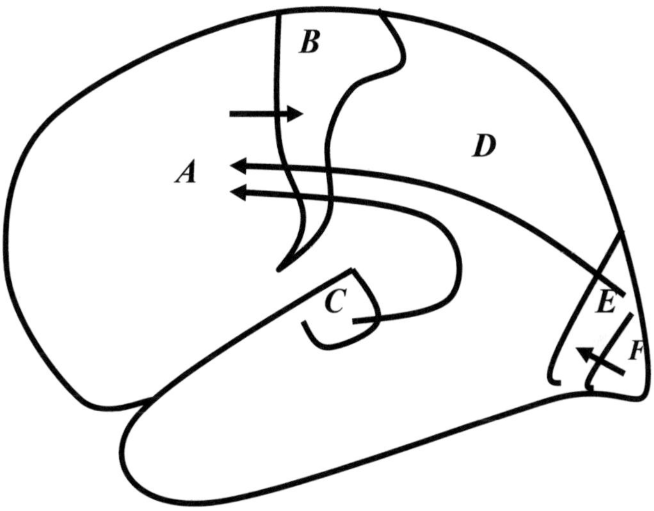

Fig. 2. Neo-associationnist model of Geschwind (1975). A, motor association cortex; B, primary motor cortex; C, Wernicke area; D, arcuate fasciculus; E, visual association cortex; F, visual cortex. Adapted from Geschwind (1975).

Tool use impairments, central to IA, are not directly concerned by this model whose primary focus is IMA. Liepmann and Maas (1907) observed that Ochs failed in some very simple object manipulations, yet could button his clothing blindfolded. They attributed this to the ability of the isolated sensory and motor cortex to do over-learned tasks without the mediation of vision. This observation corroborated previous ones indicating that LBD patients with apraxia are commonly better at demonstrating the real use of tools than at pantomiming. In line with this, Geschwind (1965) suggested that for the use of tools the pathway from primary somesthetic to primary motor cortex may be via association cortex, as in the case of connexions of other modalities to the motor system. Sparing of this pathway, as it is generally the case in LBD patients, might leave object handling totally unaffected. Given that much knowledge about tools is acquired visually, visuo-motor connections might inhibit somesthetic-motor connections, so that patients may nevertheless show some difficulties to demonstrate the actual use of tools to the sight of tools. But, as Liepmann and Maas (1907) stressed, these difficulties might be considerably reduced if patients are asked to use tools blindfolded.

3. Cognitive models of apraxia

In 1980s, there has been a renewal of interest for the study of apraxia with the emergence of cognitive models which intend to describe the different levels of processing involved in gestural production, leaving aside the issue of neuroanatomical locations. All these models share a common feature inspired from the disconnection approach of Geschwind: There would be several possible routes for producing gestures, and even the same gesture. This is the famous multiple-routes-for-action hypothesis, which diverts from Liepmann for whom there was only one mechanism. Nevertheless, unlike Geschwind, cognitive models do not conceive of apraxic manifestations as resulting from disconnections between sensorial and motor centres. They assume, as Liepmann thought, that there are several processing stages which translate sensorial codes into motor codes. In broad terms, the production of a gesture would be generally based upon conceptual processing (indirect, lexical route). But, the system would be flexible, so that conceptual processing could be bypassed (direct, non-lexical route). We discuss in more detail these models in the following lines.

3.1 Roy and Square (1985)

The model of Roy and Square (1985) is thought to rely on the operation of conceptual and production processes. The conceptual system provides an abstract representation of action relevant to limb praxis. Three types of knowledge are incorporated in this system. The first is *knowledge of objects and tools in terms of the action and functions they serve*. This kind of knowledge may have internalized linguistic referents (knowing that a knife is a piece of cutlery which can be used with a fork to eat). The second is *knowledge of actions independent of tools or objects but into which tools or objects may be incorporated*. This kind of knowledge is decontextualized, that is, associated with any particular object. People can use this practical knowledge about objects based on perceptual attributes to use tools in an unusual way (a shoe would make a good hammer). The third is *knowledge relevant to the seriation of single actions into a sequence*. Impairment of the conceptual system would lead to difficulties in pantomiming the use of tools (IMA) as well as in the actual use of objects (IA). Object substitution (e.g., using a pencil as a comb) would be one of the main manifestations of patients with defective conceptual knowledge.

While the conceptual system encompasses knowledge for action, the production system provides the mechanisms for movements. At one level, action may be directed by generalized programs representing actions and which might be of ecological importance (hammering, stirring). These programs are not specific to any particular unit (hand, foot) but can guide any of these units in the production of the action. Importantly, all of the information relevant to action would not be "in the head". Much information is also "out there" in the environment, thereby suggesting that the environment could also control the movement through bottom-up processing. Roy and Square (1985) suggested that errors in performing the sequence of movements in the sequence (omission, repetition) as well as clumsiness may be caused by impairment of the production system.

3.2 Rothi, Ochipa, and Heilman (1991)

Geschwind (1965, 1975) was opposed to the idea of specific cerebral areas in which movement formulae are stored. Nevertheless, he never tested this hypothesis. For him, the left arcuate fasciculus is dominant for visuomotor connections. And, given that these fibres pass below the left parietal cortex, deep lesions of the parietal lobe cause IMA. The corollary is that patients with damage to arcuate fasciculus and parietal lobe should encounter difficulties not only to produce gestures but also to recognize the gestures performed by others (only one form of IMA). By contrast, if the connection between the visual association cortex and the motor association cortex is relayed by movement formulae contained in the left parietal lobe, then lesions anterior to this cerebral region should cause impaired gesture production without impairment in gesture recognition.

The study of Heilman, Rothi, and Valenstein (1982) aimed at testing these predictions. They examined 20 LBD patients who were classified into four groups according to the locus of lesion (anterior vs. posterior) and whether or not they were apraxic. Apraxia was assessed by asking patients to perform 15 gestures on verbal command (12 pantomimed acts and 3 meaningful gestures such as hitchhiking). Some patients did not have a CT scan because their cerebral infarctions occurred before the advent of CT. So, they classified the subjects as fluent or non-fluent based on spontaneous speech. Because patients with fluent aphasia have generally posterior lesions and those with non-fluent aphasia have commonly anterior lesions, they used this indicator to determine the locus of lesions. Four groups were thus formed: 1, apraxic patients with anterior lesions/non-fluent aphasia; 2, apraxic patients with posterior lesions/fluent aphasia; 3, non-apraxic patients with anterior lesions/non-fluent aphasia; 4, non-apraxic patients with posterior lesions/fluent aphasia. All the patients were asked to perform a gesture discrimination test consisted of 32 trials, each containing three separate videotaped pantomimed acts. Patients were instructed to discriminate the gesture corresponding to the verbal description of the action. Only one of the three gestures was correct.

The results indicated that apraxic patients with posterior/fluent aphasia (Group 2) performed worse than the three other groups (Groups 1, 3 and 4), thereby suggesting that gesture production can be dissociated from gesture recognition and that there would be two different forms of IMA: The posterior form (impairment in both gesture recognition and gesture production: Group 2) and the anterior form (impairment in gesture production only: Group 1). These findings confirmed the hypothesis of movement formulae, which was reformulated "visuo-kinesthetic motor engrams" by Heilman et al. (1982), as well as the possible involvement of left inferior parietal lobe (supramarginal gyrus and angular gyrus) in the storage of these so-called engrams. In a subsequent study, Rothi, Heilman, and Watson (1985) asked 13 LBD patients to carry out a gesture discrimination test in which the correct gesture had to be associated with the drawing of the object. Besides corroborating the data obtained by Heilman et al. (1982), this study ruled out the possibility that the posterior type of IMA resulted from aphasia since the material used was visual and not verbal.

On the basis of these works as well as other observations of dissociation collected in the neuropsychological literature, Rothi et al. (1991) proposed a cognitive model of apraxia detailing the different processing stages required for gesture production and recognition (Figure 3). The different processing modules are presented in the following lines.

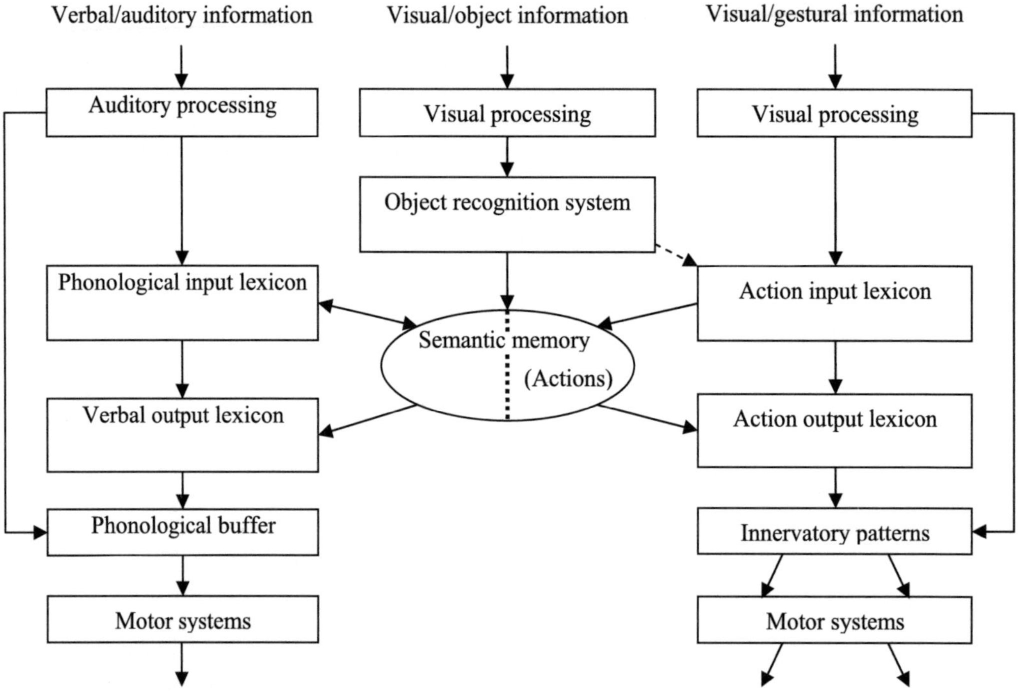

Fig. 3. Cognitive model of apraxia of Rothi et al. (1991). Note that the model is integrated into a larger cognitive architecture thought to explain language deficits. Adapted from Rothi et al. (1991).

The action-lexicon. Rothi et al. (1991) proposed the term "lexicon" to refer to the movement formulae of Liepmann (1908) and the visuokinesthetic motor engrams of Heilman et al. (1982). The model posits that input and output processing of praxis require division of the action-lexicon into an input action-lexicon (devoted to gesture recognition) and an output action-lexicon (devoted to gesture production). This distinction is supported by the fact that some patients are significantly better for recognizing or producing pantomimes on verbal command than for imitating them (Ochipa, Rothi, & Heilman, 1994). Indeed, spared gesture recognition in the presence of impaired imitation may be explained by dysfunction after access to the input action-lexicon. Moreover, given that pantomime production on verbal command is less impaired than pantomime imitation, the model assumes that spoken language might gain access to the output action-lexicon without having to be processed by the input action-lexicon.

Input modality selectivity. Rothi et al. (1991) posited that there would be selective input into the action-lexicons according to modality. This proposal is based, for example, on the observation of some patients who are able to perform gestures to command correctly, but who cannot produce visually-presented gestures (optic apraxia; see Assal & Regli, 1980). On the basis of these findings as well as other somewhat similar findings, the model suggests the existence of separate input systems for visually presented gestural information (imitation), visually presented objects (pantomime or actual tool use), and auditory presented verbal information (gestures to command).

Non-lexical action processing or direct route. In addition to a lexically based system, the model assumes that there would be a non-lexical action processing system available for the imitation of meaningful (symbolic and transitive) as well as meaningless gestures. This hypothesis is notably supported by the observation of a patient who had a selective deficit of imitation (Mehler, 1987).

Action semantics. The different stages of action processing were mainly isolated from observations of patients with IMA encountering difficulties in pantomime production or imitation. To account for IA, Rothi et al. (1991) stressed that actual tool use is dependent upon the interaction of conceptual knowledge related to tools, objects and actions, what they called action semantics. This proposal is consistent with that of Roy and Square (1985) that tool use is supported by a conceptual system (see above).

Buxbaum (2001)

For Rothi et al. (1991), damage to action lexicons should be accompanied by impairments in gesture production and comprehension and, more generally, in tasks requiring knowledge about tool manipulation. However, knowledge about tool function should not be impaired notably because this kind of knowledge would be supported by action semantics.

Buxbaum and Saffran (2002) examined this prediction with 7 aphasic patients with IMA and 6 aphasic patients without IMA. Apraxia was assessed by asking patients to perform gestures to command and on imitation (15 pantomimes and 5 symbolic gestures). Patients performed a picture-matching task in which they had to select among three tools the two tools that were the more similar to one another. In the manipulation condition, matching had to be done on the basis of similar manipulation (e.g., a typewriter and a piano are tapped with the fingertips). In the function condition, matching had to be done on the basis of similar function (e.g., a radio and a record player are used for listening music). The results indicated that apraxic patients performed worse the manipulation condition than non-apraxic patients. The opposite pattern was obtained for the function manipulation. All of the 7 apraxics and only 1 non-apraxic had lesions of the left frontoparietal cortex. The two groups did not differ in temporal lobe involvement (see also Buxbaum, Veramonti, & Schwartz, 2000b).

On the basis of these findings, Buxbaum (2001) proposed an updated version of Rothi et al.'s (1991) model, consisting of three systems (Figure 4). The first system, the dorsal action system, includes a dynamic representation of the body forming the basis for calculation of several frames of reference centred upon the body parts. Therefore, patients with "dynamic apraxia" are impaired at producing pantomime, but can use tools correctly when they are given in hand. Imitation is also defective. This apraxia could be observed after damage in the dorsal frontoparietal cortex, with involvement of the superior parietal lobe particularly likely (Buxbaum, Giovannetti, & Libon, 2000a; Heilman et al., 1982; Heilman, Rothi, Mack, Feinberg, & Watson, 1986).

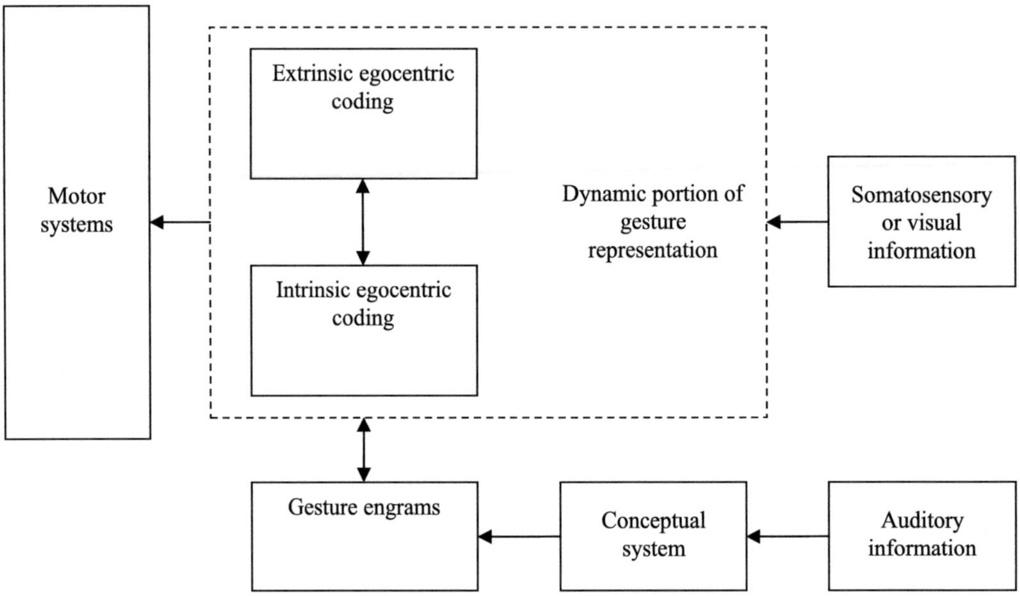

Fig. 4. Model of Buxbaum (2001). Adapted from Buxbaum (2001).

The second system, the ventral system, would include declarative, conceptual knowledge about tool function. Ventral apraxia is accompanied with difficulties with actual tool use, and more particularly in action errors revealing conceptual problems with tool knowledge (misuse, tool substitution). Gesture recognition as well as imitation would be spared. This apraxia could also be revealed by matching tasks involving knowledge about tool function (see above). Temporal lobe lesions would be critical for the occurrence of ventral apraxia (Hodges, Bozeat, Lambon Ralph, Patterson, & Spatt, 2000; Sirigu, Duhamel, & Poncet, 1991).

The third system, the central praxis system, would be specifically involved in pantomime production and recognition as well as matching tasks requiring tool manipulation (see above). This system includes gesture engrams (the action lexicons of Rothi et al., 1991) which are thought as existing at the confluence of the ventral and dorsal streams because they contain representational features (ventral system), which are themselves dependent on dynamic spatiomotor processes (dorsal system). Damage to the left inferior parietal lobe would be critical for representational apraxia (Buxbaum, Kyle, Grossman, & Coslett, 2007; Buxbaum, Kyle, & Menon, 2005; Buxbaum & Saffran, 2002; Heilman et al., 1982). For Buxbaum (2001, p. 452), gesture engrams have to be viewed as containing "the features of gestures which are invariant and critical for distinguishing a given gesture from others. For a hammering movement, for example, a broad oscillation from the elbow joint is critical, as is a clenched hand posture, and these and other similar gestural features are construed as forming the 'core' of the gesture representation".

4. Recent contribution to apraxia

The multiple-routes-for-action hypothesis is central to cognitive models of apraxia. This way of conceiving action is very heuristic by allowing the formulation of a great number of hypotheses to account for patients' difficulties. Unfortunately, this proposal is subject to a severe limitation in the interpretation of disorders. How, indeed, to demonstrate that a deficit is associated with a single process if it can always be explained by impairment at other levels? By contrast, recent works have indicated that a limited number of processes might be involved in praxis, and that they would not be parallel, but rather orthogonal. In broad terms, each process might have a specific function that could not be supported by another process. These works will be detailed in the following lines.

4.1 The role of conceptual knowledge for actual tool use

Cognitive models based on the multiple-routes-for-action hypothesis generally assign specific information to each form of conceptual knowledge. There is, however, considerable confusion about the precise role of each of these different forms, given that impairment of each of theses forms could be easily compensated. For instance, a patient with impaired conceptual knowledge about tool function may nevertheless maintain the ability to actually use tools by activating gesture engrams (Buxbaum, 2001).

In general, cognitive models distinguish, at a first level, sensorimotor, non-conceptual knowledge, about tool manipulation (i.e., visuokinesthetic motor engrams, action lexicons, gesture engrams) from conceptual/semantic knowledge[1] about tool function (Buxbaum, 2001; Rothi et al., 1991). At a second level, there is also a distinction between conceptual knowledge about the prototypical[2] use of tools (for which purpose, in which context and with which object) and knowledge containing practical information about tools and objects based on perceptual attributes (e.g., a shoe would make a good hammer) (Buxbaum, 2001; Hodges et al., 2000; Rothi et al., 1991; Roy & Square, 1985). Different tasks have been developed to assess the integrity of each of these two forms. As mentioned above, conceptual knowledge about prototypical use can be examined with picture-matching tasks in which subjects are instructed to match a tool with its usual object, its typical location or another tool that can be used to achieve the same purpose (e.g., Bozeat, Lambon Ralph, Patterson, & Hodges, 2002; Goldenberg & Spatt, 2009; Hodges, Spatt, & Patterson, 1999; Hodges et al., 2000; Osiurak et al., 2009). By contrast, practical knowledge can be evaluated by asking patients to solve mechanical problems (Goldenberg & Hagmann, 1998; Goldenberg & Spatt, 2009; Hartmann, Goldenberg, Daumüller, & Hermsdörfer, 2005) or to use familiar tools in a non-conventional way (e.g., screwing a screw with a knife) (Osiurak et al., 2007, 2008, 2009). Note that in line with the multiple-routes-for-action hypothesis, damage to one of these forms of knowledge might be compensated by the other one, and vice versa. For example, a patient showing difficulties in determining the usual function of a hammer (prototypical knowledge) might nevertheless be able to demonstrate how to use it by activating practical knowledge based on perceptual attributes. In other words, the impairment of each of these forms should not necessarily be associated with tool use disorders.

This prediction has however been invalidated by several studies indicating the existence of a strong association between practical knowledge and actual tool use. For example,

---

[1] Semantic memory is usually defined as a system that stores and retrieves information about the meaning of words, concepts and facts (Tulving, 1972; Warrington, 1975).

[2] In this chapter, we use the terms "conventional", "usual", "familiar" and "prototypical" interchangeably.

Goldenberg and Hagmann (1998) found a significant correlation in LBD patients between familiar tool use and mechanical problem solving (see also Goldenberg & Spatt, 2009; Hartmann et al., 2005; Silveri & Ciccarelli, 2009). It has also been shown that mechanical problem solving skills are often disrupted in patients with cortico-basal degeneration, who are known to exhibit severe difficulties in activities of daily life involving the use of tools[3] (Hodges et al., 1999; Spatt, Bak, Bozeat, Patterson, & Hodges, 2002). Recently, Osiurak et al. (2009) asked 20 LBD patients, 11 RBD patients and 41 healthy control subjects to perform a familiar tool use task (screwing a screw with a screwdriver) as well as a task requiring the non-conventional use of tools (screwing a screw with a knife). The findings indicated that only LBD patients encountered difficulties in the two tasks as well as a strong correlation between the two tests. While a clear-cut relationship appears to be drawn between actual tool use and practical knowledge, such a relationship has not been observed between actual tool use and prototypical knowledge. Indeed, many studies have shown that brain damage can impair actual tool use and knowledge about the prototypical use of tools (assessed with picture-matching tasks) independently from each other (Bartolo, Daumüller, Della Sala, & Goldenberg, 2007; Bozeat et al., 2002; Buxbaum, Schwartz, & Carew, 1997; Forde & Humphreys, 2000; Goldenberg & Spatt, 2009; Hodges et al., 2000; Lauro-Grotto, Piccini, & Shallice, 1997; Negri et al., 2007; Osiurak et al., 2008, 2009; Silveri & Ciccarelli, 2009).

Taken together, these findings rule out the prediction formulated above that the specific impairment of each form of conceptual knowledge (prototypical versus practical) should not cause tool use disorders. More particularly, these findings provide convincing evidence for the hypothesis that any situations involving the use of tools (actual use of familiar tools, non-conventional use of familiar tools and mechanical problem solving) might require practical but not prototypical knowledge. This conclusion raises the question as to the role of conceptual knowledge about the prototypical use for tool use.

To account for the discrepancy between these results and the predictions derived from the multiple-routes-for-action hypothesis, Buxbaum et al. (1997) suggested that prototypical knowledge may be neither necessary nor sufficient for actual tool use. Such an account is nevertheless delicate since it requires explaining why the human brain would possess knowledge that is not relevant for action. There is another way to interpret these findings, but this implies ruling out the multiple-routes-for-action hypothesis by considering that each form of knowledge has an assigned function. In this way, Osiurak et al. (2008, 2009, 2010, 2011) have suggested that practical knowledge - what they called "technical reasoning" - would be specifically devoted to the formation of representations about the possible physical actions on the world (see also McCloskey, 1983; Penn, Holyoak, & Povinelli, 2008). By contrast, prototypical knowledge, as any semantic knowledge, would enable people to determine the usage of tools, that is, in which context, in which location or with which object a given tool is commonly employed. This second form of knowledge would be particularly useful for adapting oneself to social usages in knowing, for example, that a toothbrush is appropriate for cleaning teeth and not shoes or that Japanese people use sticks and not forks and knives to eat.

[3] It is noteworthy that we do not refer here to the difficulties observed in actual tool use because of motor apraxia, but those difficulties that are due to conceptual impairment and which appear later in the disease (see below).

In line with this proposal, it can be predicted that patients with a selective semantic deficit and, as a result, impaired prototypical knowledge, should meet difficulties to demonstrate how tools presented in isolation (pantomime, use of tools in isolation) are usually used. Recently, we brought evidence for this prediction by describing the case of the patient MJC who had a severe semantic impairment (matching picture tasks) following closed head injury (Osiurak et al., 2008). This patient was unable to demonstrate the use of tools presented in isolation. Very interestingly, MJC used almost systematically the desk to show the use of tools, as she attempted to bring out mechanical relationships from the desk and the tools. For instance, she used a key to for scrapping the chamfered edge of the wooden desk or a screwdriver as a gimlet, adding that "one can make a hole with it". Nevertheless, MJC performed normally when asked to use tools presented with their corresponding objects and was even able to use tools in a non-conventional way to the extent that these tools were present with a given object (see above). Somewhat similar strategies were also reported by Sirigu et al. (1991) who described a patient (FB) with bitemporal lobe lesions caused by herpetic encephalitis. FB was unable to recognize many familiar tools and objects, but could describe how these tools could be manipulated. For instance, when asked to identify a nail clipper, he said that "it can attach several sheets of paper together. You turn the piece on the top and tip it back...You press and it maintains them" (Sirigu et al., 1991, p. 2566). Recent works on patients with semantic dementia have also shown a strong association between semantic picture matching tasks and the use of isolated tools (Hodges et al., 2000; Silveri & Ciccarelli, 2009).

In sum, these findings reveal that the actual use of tools presented in isolation - and therefore production of pantomimes to command or to the sight of tools - poses serious problems to patients with semantic impairment[4]. Interestingly, these patients tend to employ a compensatory strategy consisting in using the immediate environment in order to bring out possible actions which are, as a result, not necessarily the actions usually carried out with the tools. This can be easily explained by the preservation of practical knowledge. Of course, we are not saying that the human brain would contain semantic, prototypical knowledge whose main purpose would be to enable patients to show how an isolated tool can be used. As discussed above, prototypical knowledge may be particularly relevant for adapting oneself to social situations, but also to retrieve tools that are not immediately present to the senses. After all, knowledge about the fact that nails can generally be found in a workshop enables people to seek the tool necessary for completing the current action in the appropriate place. But, in the clinical context, the involvement of prototypical knowledge might be more pronounced when patients are asked to demonstrate the use of isolated tools. Note that this also requires examining whether the performance improves when the corresponding object is given. If such improvement occurs along with difficulties in semantic picture matching tasks, then the hypothesis of a selective semantic impairment can be reasonably formulated.

The evaluation of semantic disorders we propose here differs from the classical, cognitive approach which focuses on the type of errors committed by patients to specify the nature of the deficit (e.g., content errors would be specific to semantic impairment). However, we think that this way of addressing apraxia is delicate because it is generally very hard to

[4] Note that the distinction we make here between the use of tools in isolation versus with the corresponding object does not appear in the cognitive models discussed above.

distinguish content errors from other types of errors. Our way of assessing the impairment is simpler and is based on the conjunction of the deficits observed in a patient on several different tasks (Table 1). Moreover, it is noteworthy that semantic impairment could be found more frequently in patients with bilateral or left temporal lobe lesions, that is, in patients with cortical degeneration (semantic dementia or Alzheimer's disease) or after vascular lesions of these areas.

Task	Production system (motor apraxia)	Conceptual system		
		Prototypical knowledge	Practical knowledge	Topographical knowledge about body parts
Sequence of finger movements	Impaired	Normal	Normal	Normal
Functional picture matching	Normal	Impaired	Normal	Normal
Use of isolated tools	Impaired manipulation	Impaired	Impaired	Normal
Use of tools with corresponding objects	Impaired manipulation	Normal	Impaired	Normal
Selection of the correct tools and use of it with a given object	Impaired manipulation	Normal	Impaired	Normal
Mechanical problem solving	Impaired manipulation	Normal	Impaired	Normal
Imitation of meaningless hand postures	Quasi-normal	Normal	Normal	Impaired
Imitation of meaningless finger postures	Impaired	Normal	Normal	Normal

The distinction we make here between production system versus conceptual system is not based on the different cognitive models presented in this chapter since none of them suggests that the conceptual system would contain prototypical knowledge, practical knowledge and topographical knowledge about body parts. Rather, this distinction corresponds to a synthesis of the works presented here.

Table 1. Examination of apraxia

With regard to the neuroanatomical loci of damage associated with impaired practical knowledge, it is interesting to note that many works have pointed out that anomalous tool use is generally present in patients with large bilateral or left fronto-parieto-temporal lobe lesions (Fukutake, 2008; Rumiati, Zanini, Vorano, & Shallice, 2001), even though it is not systematic (Halsband et al., 2000). In this study, five patients with circumscribed lesions of the left parietal cortex did not encounter any difficulty to use tools. In fact, De Renzi and Lucchelli (1988) had already indicated that IA was not systematically present in patients with parietal lobe lesions. More recently, Goldenberg and Hagmann (1998) examined the ability to use tools in LBD patients. They did not find any association between tool use performance and specific brain areas. In a more recent study, Goldenberg and Spatt (2009) asked 38 LBD patients to perform a familiar tool use test as well as a mechanical problem solving task. The correlational analysis between the scores and the lesional sites indicated that left parietal and frontal, but not temporal areas played a significant role in the two tasks. In total, it appears that the left parietal lobe might store practical knowledge, although more extended lesions of the left hemisphere and even of the right hemisphere could be necessary for the emergence of clinically observable difficulties. So, impaired practical knowledge might be more frequent in diseases causing lesions in these areas (stroke, some degenerative diseases such as the cortico-basal degeneration at advanced stage or Alzheimer's disease).

4.2 Imitation of meaningless gestures

The multiple-routes-for-action hypothesis assumes that there would be a non-lexical, direct route between early visual centres and motor centres. This proposal has been supported by observations of patients with a visuo-imitative apraxia, that is, a specific or at least more pronounced deficit of imitation of meaningless gestures (Mehler, 1987; Ochipa et al., 1994). Several studies have however questioned the existence of this direct route.

Goldenberg (1995) asked 35 LBD patients, 20 RBD patients and 20 healthy subjects to imitate meaningless hand postures as well as to replicate the gestures on a life-sized manikin. All the postures involved the face. The results indicated that LBD patients performed dramatically worse than RBD patients and controls on both tests. In another study, Goldenberg and Hagmann (1997) reported two patients (LK and EN) with left inferior parietal lobe lesions (angular gyrus) who were also severely impaired at imitating these postures as well as replicating on the manikin. On the basis of these findings, Goldenberg and Hagmann (1997; see also Goldenberg, 1997) suggested that imitation of meaningless hand postures is not based on a direct route between perception and action, but might be rather mediated by general topographical knowledge about the human body.

Goldenberg and Hagmann (1997) also developed a task of imitation of meaningless finger postures and showed that EN but not LK failed this test. This distinction was quite surprising given that until this work no neuropsychologist had focused on a possible distinction between imitation of hand versus finger postures. In fact, the evaluation was generally based on a composite score obtained from the two conditions (e.g., De Renzi, Motti, & Nichelli, 1980). Goldenberg (1999) examined 26 LBD patients, 21 RBD patients and 17 healthy subjects on imitation as well as matching of meaningless hand and finger postures. He found that LBD patients performed worse than RBD patients for hand posture imitation and matching, whereas the opposite pattern was observed for finger postures. So, he concluded that imitation and matching of hand postures would be based on topographical knowledge about body parts and would involve the left parietal lobe. Indeed, given that the hand is in contact with the face, the patient does not see the posture he/she is carrying out. So, the ability to execute such gestures needs knowledge about body parts and notably the face (knowing that the extremity of the hand must be in contact with the nose implies being able to distinguish the nose from other parts of the face). By contrast, imitation and matching of finger postures would be based on visuo-spatial skills supported by the right posterior cerebral hemisphere. Indeed, the reproduction of finger postures requires visual guidance in order to represent the position of each finger relative to the others. The involvement of topographical knowledge about body parts is here largely limited. These conclusions were corroborated by more recent neuroimaging studies conducted in healthy subjects (Hermsdörfer et al., 2001; see also Goldenberg, Laimgruber, & Hermsdörfer, 2001).

Besides challenging the relevance of the multiple-routes-for-action hypothesis and notably the existence of the non-lexical, direct route, these findings more generally challenged the interest of proposing a unique cognitive model of apraxia accounting for tool use and imitation impairment. Note also that the works by Goldenberg, as those mentioned above about the distinction between the use of tools in isolation versus with the corresponding object, shed a new light on the evaluation of apraxia, in stressing that even if situations may appear quite similar, subtle modifications in the material used can lead to observe very different disorders. Consequently, the distinction demonstrated by Goldenberg between finger versus hand postures must be taken into consideration in the clinical assessment of apraxia (Table 1). Finally, it is noteworthy that the association observed by Goldenberg between imitation of meaningless hand postures and the left inferior parietal lobe is inconsistent with the cognitive models discussed above. Indeed, in those models, the left inferior parietal region is thought to contain gesture engrams. Yet, other studies have confirmed the relationship obtained by Goldenberg. For instance, Haaland, Harrington, and Knight (2000) found that patients who were impaired at imitating meaningless hand postures generally had left inferior parietal lobe lesions (supramarginal gyrus and angular gyrus). Moreover, they also reported that errors concerning the position of the hand relative to the face were only present in patients with parietal lobe lesions whereas the errors concerning the position of the fingers relative to the others were rather present in patients with frontal damage and in only 60% of the patients with parietal lobe lesions (see also Goldenberg & Karnath, 2006).

4.3 Pantomime production, actual tool use and gesture engrams

The cognitive models discussed above, with the exception of Roy and Square's (1985), suggest that knowledge about tool manipulation are supported by gesture engrams. Quite surprisingly, damage to these engrams would not cause significant difficulties in actual tool use, because physical constraints inherent to tools and objects could be sufficient to guide the utilization. The corollary is that damage to gesture engrams mainly affects the production of pantomimes. If it can be thought that the clinical tasks, even if they are often not ecological, may be relevant for revealing impairment, it can nevertheless seem somewhat surprising to consider that the major role of these representations would be to support pantomime production, namely, a situation people meet very rarely in real life. In order to solve this theoretical curiosity, it has been suggested that damage to gesture engrams might cause subtle manipulation errors during actual tool use and that these errors might occur conjointly with the errors observed in pantomime production (Clark et al., 1994; Rothi et al., 1991). In line with this prediction, Clark et al. (1994; see also Poizner, Clark, Merians, & Macauley, 1995) asked 3 apraxic LBD patients to carry out the action "slicing bread" in 4 conditions: No cues (verbal command only), object present (bread), tool present (knife) and both object and tool present (bread and knife). Gestures were recorded and submitted to kinematic analyses. Results indicated that patients showed disturbances in planning the movement of the hand in space across the 4 conditions. These findings were thought as providing evidence for the existence of gesture engrams.

These results are however to be considered with caution because of several methodological limitations. For example, the size of the patient sample was relatively weak and could not allow the use of statistical correlations between the errors observed in the 4 conditions. More recently, Hermsdörfer, Hentze, and Goldenberg. (2006; see also Goldenberg, Hentze, & Hermsdörfer, 2004) replicated this experiment by asking 9 apraxic LBD patients to carry out the action "sawing a piece of wood" in 3 conditions: Pantomime (visual presentation of the saw), pantomime with a bar shaped like the handle of the saw, and actual sawing. Gestures were recorded and submitted to kinematic analyses. Results revealed that, patients executed large proportions of their pantomiming movements in an incorrect direction away from the appropriate anteroposterior direction. The availability of the handle-like bar did not improve performance. During actual use, patients moved with moderately decreased velocity. However, this deficit was not related to the errors in movement direction characteristic of pantomiming, suggesting that pantomime and actual tool use are dictated by different requirements and constraints. In broad terms, unlike Clark et al. (1994), manipulation errors during actual tool use do not occur conjointly with the errors observed in pantomime production.

On the basis of these findings, it appears that the gesture engram hypothesis fails to explain how people use tools or produce pantomimes. Again, that these models primarily focus on the ability to perform pantomimes may appear somewhat surprising as people carry out such actions quite occasionally in real life as compared to actual tool use. In fact, in line with the distinction made above between prototypical versus practical knowledge, another interpretation can be offered with regard to pantomime production. The demonstration by pantomime, like any other tool use situation, requires technical reasoning (see above) to create a representation of the action (the use of the tool). Unlike actual tool use, however, people have to carry out actions, while some of the components (the tool and/or the object) are not available to the senses. So, in a way similar to the use of isolated tools (see above), people have to form representations of these components from semantic/conceptual memory, putting high demands on storage and elaboration because the performance can be guided and controlled only with reference to these representations (Goldenberg, Hartmann, & Schlott, 2003; Roy & Hall, 1992). Moreover, in the context of pantomime, after the representation of the use is produced, it is still necessary to keep it in mind to convert into a pantomime the shape, movement and position of the acting hand via an affordance-perception process (Bartolo, Cubelli, Della Sala, & Drei, 2003; Goldenberg et al., 2003; Roy & Hall, 1992). In short, the demonstration by pantomime would be a non-routine, creative task, consisting in the creation and the temporary storage of a representation of the use which then guides the movement. Note also that in line with the gesture engram hypothesis, disturbance in pantomime production should be accompanied by lesions of the left inferior parietal cortex. However, it has been demonstrated that it remains relatively hard to specify precise brain localisations associated with the performance of pantomime production (Alexander, Baker, Naeser, Kaplan, & Palumbo, 1992; Goldenberg, 2003; Goldenberg et al., 2003; see also Goldenberg, 2009).

To sum up, performance in pantomime tasks remain hard to interpret because of the involvement of a high number of cognitive processes. This may explain why pantomime production is frequently impaired after lesions in various areas of the left hemisphere (Goldenberg, 2003). Moreover, even if the use of three-dimensional motion recording systems or the development of procedure based on video-recording and multiple-judge techniques have allowed neuropsychologists to improve the measurement of movements in an objective way, these procedures remain very far from the reality of clinicians who evaluate patients' performance on the basis of their own experience and intuition (Le Gall, 1992: Poeck, 1986). So, we advise employing pantomime tasks with caution and parsimony and we favour the use of other tasks involving the actual use of tools or imitation of meaningless postures.

4.4 The independance of motor apraxia

So far, we have focused on the conceptual facet of apraxic manifestations. In this section, we put an emphasis on "motor apraxia" also called "melo-kinetic apraxia" or "limb-kinetic apraxia", corresponding with the other facet of the syndrome (production).

Kleist (1907) was the first to describe the loss of hand and finger dexterity resulting from inability to isolate individual innervation. This lack of dexterity is generally confined to hand and finger movements contralateral to the lesion, regardless of the hemisphere which is damaged. The deficit can be distinguished from paresis because of preservation of power and sensation. Nevertheless, movements are awkward. Fruitless attempts commonly precede erroneous movements, which are frequently contaminated by extraneous movements. Importantly, the deficit is consistent, showing the same degree in activities of daily life. In other words, there is no voluntary-automatic dissociation. For Kleist (1907), this disorder reveals damage to innervatory patterns acquired with experience. He called this deficit "innervatory apraxia".

Denny-Brown (1958) provided an original way of conceiving of motor apraxia in distinguishing "frontal, magnetic apraxia" from "parietal, repellent apraxia". The first type is characterised by prominence and persistence of instinctive grasping of the hands, the mouth and even the feet when they make contact or even merely when they are close to any object. Object manipulation can be impaired because patients do not open the hand wide enough when they take hold of an object. The magnetic, exploratory aspect of this behaviour in relation to the environment would be managed by the parietal cortex, released by frontal and temporal lobe lesions. The second type is characterized by avoiding reaction and levitation of the extremities. Similarly, object manipulation may be impaired because of overextension when patients attempt to pick up of grasp objects. The repellent bias to behaviour would be determined by a strip of cerebral cortex in the premotor region and released by parietal lobe damage. These two types of apraxia are unilateral and can generate problems in bimanual activities or in tasks requiring the coordination of the two "hemi-bodies". Denny-Brown stressed the functional independence of these forms of apraxia from conceptual skills. He reported, for instance, the observation of a patient unable to correctly grasp a pair of scissors, but could cut up a piece of paper if it was helped to correctly grasp the pair of scissors.

Interestingly, this observation points out the severe difficulties that patients with motor apraxia can encounter when they have to carry out distal movements involving a precise positioning of the fingers. In another study, Sirigu et al. (1995) also reported disturbances in the ability to adequately grasp tools to actually use them in a patient with bilateral superior parietal lobe lesions. Nevertheless, when the examiner helped this patient to correctly grasp the tool, the demonstration was performed properly.

Motor apraxia has received a resurgence of interest in recent years with the study of patients with cortico-basal degeneration. This disease is characterized by an akinetic-rigid syndrome accompanied by asymmetric, lateralizing cortical signs including alien limb behaviour, sensory loss and apraxia (Gibb, Luthert, & Marsden, 1989; see also Zadikoff & Lang, 2005). Imaging studies have revealed the presence of frontoparietal cortical atrophy, which is most notable contralateral to the most severely affected side. Two types of apraxia are present in patients with cortico-basal degeneration: Motor apraxia and IMA. Some patients can also show signs of IA, but this kind of apraxia would appear later in the disease (Gibb et al., 1989; Leiguarda, Lees, Merello, Starkstein, & Marsden, 1994). While a significant number of patients have a bilateral IMA (pantomime to command or on imitation; see Zadikoff & Lang, 2005), IMA is generally unilateral at early stages of the disease. This questions the independence of IMA from motor apraxia given that this latter is specifically unilateral.

As Kleist (1907) suggested, the severity of motor apraxia is more pronounced in distal than proximal movements, and can be readily observed in tasks requiring the coordination of finger movements in actual tool use or imitation of gestures (Leiguarda & Marsden, 2000; Zadikoff & Lang, 2005). One effective way of assessing motor apraxia is to ask patients to carry out sequence of finger movements (1-4-2-4). Nevertheless, this task as any other task is certainly not supported only on the production system and can also be failed, for example, by patients with visuo-spatial deficits (see above). So, the best way to determine the presence of motor apraxia remains to examine whether impairment is constant across the tasks. For example, in order to isolate motor apraxia from other disorders during tool use, we advise first examining whether the patient does not have impaired practical knowledge by asking him/her first to select among several tools (hammer, key, saw) the appropriate one to be used with a given object (nail). If the choice is correct, then this implies that the patient is still able to correctly reason about the physical properties of tools and objects and, as a result, to form an appropriate representation of the action. And, if the patient shows severe difficulties to manipulate the tool to show its use with the object, then it is very likely that the patient has a motor apraxia. In sum, we agree with Foix (1916) who challenged the idea that tool use impairment is based on damage to motor representations. For him, IA was due to a general intellectual deficit and motor apraxia was the only form of apraxia. For us, IA was rather due to the inability to do technical reasoning (see above).

5. Conclusion

As mentioned above, the study of apraxia has been subject to intense debate, particularly with regard to its independence from other cognitive processes. The emergence of cognitive models has contributed to the idea that damage to sensorimotor representations (gesture engrams) would be central to apraxia and particularly IMA. Recent findings have however shed a new light on this issue, suggesting that the debate is far from being resolved. As Foix (1916) and Morlass (1928) thought, there might be only one form of apraxia, that is, motor apraxia, the other types of apraxia being nothing else than the manifestations of conceptual disorders in gesture production. After all, when a patient fails an episodic memory test by pointing the wrong word, this gestural error is not characterized as apraxic. Likewise, a patient who is impaired at performing the Tower of London Test may also be considered as expressing manipulation errors. Yet, nobody would consider that this patient is apraxic. So, the question remains to understand what the arguments are leading neuropsychologists to still think that the difficulties observed in actual tool use is necessarily due to damage to sensorimotor representations.

The framework we offer here allows renewing the assessment of disorders which are generally viewed as apraxia. We have given examples concerning the evaluation of practical versus prototypical knowledge. Importantly, the evaluation we advise lies in the principle that it is necessary to escape from the assessment of the quality of movements per se, and rather to view disorders as the manifestation of a deficit that is constant across the tasks. This is not to say that the observation of the gestures executed by patients do not provide any information concerning the disease. If the difficulties are indeed constant across several gestural tasks, then it is very likely that the patient has a motor apraxia (Table 1). But, expected from motor apraxia, the focus must not be placed on the movement executed but rather on the nature of the task which is failed (actual tool use, imitation).

6. Acknowledgments

This work was supported by grants from ANR (Agence Nationale pour la Recherche; Project Démences et Utilisation d'Outils/Dementia and Tool Use, N°ANR 2011 MALZ 006 03) to both authors.

7. References

Alexander, M. P., Baker, E., Naeser, M. A., Kaplan, E., & Palumbo, C. (1992). Neuropsychological and neuroanatomic dimensions of ideomotor apraxia. *Brain, 115*, 87-107.

Assal, G., & Regli, F. (1980). Syndrome de déconnexion visuo-verbale et visuo-gestuelle. Aphasie optique et apraxie optique. *Revue Neurologique, 136*, 365–376.

Bartolo, A., Cubelli, R., Della Sala, S., & Drei, S. (2003). Pantomimes are special gestures which rely on working memory. *Brain and Cognition, 53*, 483–494.

Bartolo, A., Daumüller, M., Della Sala, S., & Goldenberg, G. (2007). Relationship between object-related gestures and the fractionated object knowledge system. *Behavioural Neurology, 18*, 143–147.

Bozeat, S., Lambon Ralph, M. A., Patterson, K., & Hodges, J. R. (2002). When objects lose their meaning: What happens to their use? *Cognitive, Affective and Behavioral Neurosciences, 2*, 236–251.

Buxbaum, L. J. (2001). Ideomotor Apraxia: A call to action. *Neurocase, 7*, 445–448.

Buxbaum, L. J., Giovannetti, T., & Libon, D. (2000a). The role of the dynamic body schema in praxis: Evidence from primary progressive apraxia. *Brain and Cognition, 44*, 166–191.

Buxbaum, L. J., Kyle, K. M, Grossman, M., & Coslett, H. B. (2007). Left inferior parietal representations for skilled hand-object interactions: Evidence from stroke and corticobasal degeneration. *Cortex, 43*, 411–423.

Buxbaum, L. J., Kyle, K. M., & Menon, R. (2005). On beyond mirror neurons: Internal representations subserving imitation and recognition of skilled object-related actions in humans. *Cognitive Brain Research, 25*, 226–239.

Buxbaum, L. J., & Saffran, E.M. (2002). Knowledge of object manipulation and object function: Dissociations in apraxic and nonapraxic subjects. *Brain and Language, 82*, 179–199.

Buxbaum, L. J., Schwartz, M. F., & Carew, T. G. (1997). The role of memory in object use. *Cognitive Neuropsychology, 14*, 219–254.

Buxbaum, L. J., Veramonti, T., & Schwartz, M. F. (2000b). Function and manipulation tool knowledge in apraxia: Knowing "what for" but not "how". *Neurocase, 6*, 83–97.

Clark, M. A., Merians, A. S., Kothari, A., Poizner, H., Macauley, B., Rothi, L. J. G., & Heilman, K. M. (1994). Spatial planning deficits in limb apraxia. *Brain, 117*, 1093–1106.

De Renzi, E. (1989). Apraxia. In F. Boller, & J. Grafman (Eds.), *Handbook of neuropsychology* (pp. 245–263). Amsterdam: Elsevier.

De Renzi, E., & Lucchelli, F. (1988). Ideational apraxia. *Brain, 111*, 1173–1185.

De Renzi, E., Motti, F., & Nichelli, P. (1980). Imitating gestures: A quantitative approach to ideomotor apraxia. *Archives of Neurology, 37*, 6–18.

Denny-Brown, D. (1958). The nature of apraxia. *The Journal of Nervous and Mental Disease, 126*, 9–32.

Foix, C. (1916). Contribution à l'étude de l'apraxie idéomotrice. *Revue Neurologique, 29*, 285–298.

Forde, E.M.E., & Humphreys, G.W. (2000). The role of semantic knowledge and working memory in everyday tasks. *Brain and Cognition, 44*, 214–252.

Fukutake, T. (2008). Apraxia of tool use: An autopsy case of biparietal infarction. *European Neurology, 49*, 45–52.

Geschwind, N. (1965). Disconnection syndrome in animal and man. *Brain, 88*, 585–644.

Geschwind, N. (1975). The apraxias. Neural mechanisms of disorders of learned movement. *American Scientist, 63*, 188–195.

Geschwind, N, & Kaplan, E. (1962). A human cerebral disconnection syndrome. *Neurology, 12*, 675–685.

Gibb, W. R. G., Luthert, P. J., & Marsden, C. D. (1989). Corticobasal degeneration. *Brain, 112*, 1171–1192.

Gogol, N. (1873). *Ein Beitrag zur lehre von der Aphasie*. Breslau, Inaugural Dissertation.

Goldenberg, G. (1995). Imitating gestures and manipulating a manikin. The representation of the human body in ideomotor apraxia. *Neuropsychologia, 33*, 63–72.

Goldenberg, G. (1997). Disorders of body perception. In T. E. Feinberg & M. J. Farah (Eds.), *Behavioural Neurology and Neuropsychology* (pp. 289–296). New York: Mac Graw-Hill.

Goldenberg, G. (1999). Matching and imitation of hand and finger postures in patients with damage in the left or right hemispheres. *Neuropsychologia, 37*, 559–566.

Goldenberg, G. (2003). Pantomime of object use: a challenge to cerebral localization of cognitive function. *NeuroImage, 20*, 101–106.

Goldenberg, G. (2009). Apraxia and the parietal lobes. *Neuropsychologia, 47*, 1449–1559.

Goldenberg, G., & Hagmann, S. (1997). The meaning of meaningless gestures: A study of visuo-imitative apraxia. *Neuropsychologia, 35*, 333–341.

Goldenberg, G., & Hagmann, S. (1998). Tool use and mechanical problem solving in apraxia. *Neuropsychologia, 36*, 581–589.

Goldenberg, G., Hartmann, K., & Schlott, I. (2003). Defective pantomime of object use in left brain damage: Apraxia or asymbolia? *Neuropsychologia, 41*, 1565–1573.

Goldenberg, G., Hentze, S., & Hermsdörfer, J. (2004). The effect of tactile feedback on pantomime of tool use in apraxia. *Neurology, 63*, 1863–1867.

Goldenberg, G., & Karnath, H. O. (2006). The neural basis of imitation is body part specific. *The Journal of Neurosciences, 26*, 6282–6287.

Goldenberg, G., Laimgruber, K., & Hermsdörfer, J. (2001). Imitation of gestures by disconnected hemispheres. *Neuropsychologia, 39,* 1432–1443.

Goldenberg, G., & Spatt, J. (2009). The neural basis of tool use. *Brain, 132,* 1645–1655.

Haaland, K. Y., Harrington, D. L., & Knight, R. T. (2000). Neural representations of skilled movement. *Brain, 123,* 2306–2313.

Halsband, U., Weyers, M., Schmitt, J., Binkofski, F., Grützner, G., & Freund, H. J. (2000). Recognition and imitation of pantomimed motor acts after unilateral parietal and premotor lesions: A perspective on apraxia. *Neuropsychologia, 39,* 200–216.

Hartmann, K., Goldenberg, G., Daumüller, M., & Hermsdörfer, J. (2005). It takes the whole brain to make a cup of coffee: The neuropsychology of naturalistic actions involving technical devices. *Neuropsychologia, 43,* 625–637.

Heilman, K. M., Rothi, L. J. G., Mack, L., Feinberg, T., & Watson, R. T. (1986). Apraxia after superior parietal lesions. *Cortex, 32,* 141–150.

Heilman, K. M., Rothi, L. J., & Valenstein, E. (1982). Two forms of ideomotor apraxia. *Neurology, 22,* 342–346.

Hermsdörfer, J., Goldenberg, G., Wachsmuth, C., Conrad, B., Ceballos-Baumann, A. O., Bartenstein, P., Schwaiger, M., & Boecker, H. (2001). Cortical correlates of gesture processing: Clues to the cerebral mechanisms underlying apraxia during the imitation of meaningless gestures. *NeuroImage, 14,* 149–161.

Hermsdörfer, J., Hentze, S., & Goldenberg, G. (2006). Spatial and kinematic features of apraxic movement depend on the mode of execution. *Neuropsychologia, 44,* 1642–1652.

Hodges, J. R., Bozeat, S., Lambon Ralph, M. A., Patterson, K., & Spatt, J. (2000). The role of knowledge in object use: Evidence from semantic dementia. *Brain, 123,* 1913–1925.

Hodges, J. R., Spatt, J., & Patterson, K. (1999). "What" and "how": Evidence for the dissociation of object knowledge and mechanical problem-solving skills in the human brain. *Proceeding of the National Academy of Sciences of the United States of America, 96,* 9444–9448.

Jackson, H. (1866). Notes on the physiology and pathology of language. *Brain, 38,* 48–58.

Kleist, K. (1907). Kortikale (innervatorische) Apraxie. *Jahrbuch für Psychiatrie und Neurologie, 28,* 46–112.

Lauro-Grotto, R. Piccini, C., & Shallice, T. (1997). Modality-specific operations in semantic dementia. *Cortex, 33,* 593–622.

Le Gall, D. (1992). Apraxies idéo-motrice et idéatoire: Revue critique de la littérature. *Revue de Neuropsychologie, 2,* 325–371.

Leiguarda, R. C., Lees, A. J., Merello, S., Starkstein, S., & Marsden, C. D. (1994). The nature of apraxia in corticobasal degeneration. *Journal of Neurology, Neurosurgery, and Psychiatry, 57,* 455–459.

Leiguarda, R. C., & Marsden, C. D. (2000). Limb apraxias. Higher-order disorders of sensorimotor integration. *Brain, 123,* 860–879.

Liepmann, H. (1900). Das Krankheitsbild der Apraxie ("Motorischen Asymbolie") auf Grund eines Falles von einseitiger Apraxie. *Monatschrift für Psychiatrie und Neurologie, 8,* 15–44.

Liepmann, H. (1908). *Drei aufsatze aus dem apraxiegebiet*. Berlin: Karger.

Liepmann, H. (1920). Apraxie. *Ergebnisse der gesamten Medizin, 1,* 516–540.

Liepmann, H., & Maas, O. (1907). Fall von linksseitiger Agraphie und Apraxie bei rechtsseitiger Lahmung. *Zeitschrift für Psychologie und Neurologie, 10,* 214-227.
McCloskey, M. (1983). Intuitive physics. *Scientific American, 248,* 395–400.
Mehler, F.M. (1987). Visuo-imitative apraxia. *Neurology, 37,* 129.
Morlaas, J. (1928). *Contribution à l'étude de l'apraxie.* Paris: Legrand.
Negri, G. A. L., Rumiati, R. I., Zadini, A., Ukmar, M., Mahon, B. Z., & Caramazza, A. (2007). What is the role of motor stimulation in action and object recognition? Evidence from apraxia. *Cognitive Neuropsychology, 24,* 795–816.
Ochipa, C., Rothi, L. J. G, & Heilman, K. M. (1994). Conduction apraxia. *Journal of Neurology, Neurosurgery and Psychiatry, 57,* 1241-1244.
Osiurak, F., Aubin, G., Allain, P., Jarry, C., Richard, I., & Le Gall, D. (2008). Object usage and object utilization. A single-case study. *Neurocase, 14,* 169-183.
Osiurak, F., Jarry, C., Allain, P., Aubin, G., Etcharry-Bouyx, F., Richard, I., Bernard, I., & Le Gall, D. (2009). Unusual use of objects after unilateral brain damage. The technical reasoning model. *Cortex, 45,* 769-783.
Osiurak, F., Jarry, C., Allain, P., Aubin, G., Etcharry-Bouyx, F., Richard, I., & Le Gall, D. (2007). Des troubles praxiques aux troubles techniques. Une étude de deux cas. *Revue de Neuropsychologie, 17,* 231-259.
Osiurak, F., Jarry, C., & Le Gall, D. (2010). Grasping the affordances, understanding the reasoning. Toward a dialectical theory of human tool use. *Psychological Review, 117,* 517-540.
Osiurak, F., Jarry, C., & Le Gall, D. (2011). Re-examining the gesture engram hypothesis. New perspectives on apraxia of tool use. *Neuropsychologia, 49,* 299-312.
Penn, D. C., Holyoak, K. J., & Povinelli, D. J. (2008). Darwin's mistake: Explaining the discontinuity between human and nonhuman minds. *Behavioral and Brain Sciences, 31,* 109-130.
Pick, A. (1905). *Studien über motorische Apraxie und ihre nahe stehende Erscheinungen.* Leipzig: Deuticke.
Poeck, K. (1986). The clinical examination for motor apraxia. *Neuropsychologia, 24,* 129-134.
Poizner, H., Clark, M., Merians, A. S., & Macauley, B. (1995). Joint coordination deficits in limb apraxia. *Brain, 118,* 227-242.
Rothi, L. J., Heilman, K. M., & Watson, R. T. (1985). Pantomime comprehension and ideomotor apraxia. *Journal of Neurology, Neurosurgery and Psychiatry, 48,* 207-210.
Rothi, L. J. G., Ochipa, C., & Heilman, K. M. (1991). A cognitive neuropsychological model of limb praxis. *Cognitive Neuropsychology, 8,* 443-458.
Roy, E. A., & Hall, C. (1992). Limb apraxia. A process approach. In P. Luc, & E. Digby (Eds.), *Vision and motor control* (pp. 261-282). Amsterdam: Elsevier.
Roy, E. A., & Square, P. A. (1985). Common considerations in the study of limb, verbal and oral apraxia. In E. A. Roy (Ed.), *Neuropsychological studies of apraxia and related disorders* (pp. 111-161). Amsterdam: Elsevier.
Rumiati, R., Zanini, S., Vorano, L., & Shallice, T. (2001). A form of ideational apraxia as a selective deficit of contention scheduling. *Cognitive Neuropsychology, 18,* 617-642.
Silveri, M. C., & Ciccarelli, N. (2009). Semantic memory in object use. *Neuropsychologia, 47,* 2634-2641.
Sirigu, A., Cohen, L., Duhamel, J. -R., Pillon, B., Dubois, B., & Agid, Y. (1995). A selective impairment of hand posture for object utilization in apraxia. *Cortex, 31,* 41-55.

Sirigu, A., Duhamel, J. -R., & Poncet, M. (1991). The role of sensorimotor experience in object recognition. *Brain, 114,* 2555–2573.

Spatt, J., Bak, T., Bozeat, S., Patterson, K., & Hodges, J. R. (2002). Apraxia, mechanical problem solving and semantic knowledge: Contributions to object usage in corticobasal degeneration. *Journal of Neurology, 249,* 601–608.

Steinthal, H. (1871). *Abriss der Sprachwissenschaft.* Berlin.

Tulving, E. (1972). Episodic and semantic memory. In E. Tulving & W. Donaldson (Eds.), *Organization of memory* (pp. 381–403). New York: Academic Press.

Warrington, E. K. (1975). The selective impairment of semantic memory. *Quarterly Journal of Experimental Psychology, 27,* 635–657.

Zadikoff, C., & Lang, A. E. (2005). Apraxia in movement disorders. *Brain, 128,* 1480–1497.

5

Neurocognitive Deficits in Patients with Obstructive Sleep Apnea Syndrome (OSAS)

Georgia Andreou, Filippos Vlachos and Konstantinos Makanikas
Department of Special Education, University of Thessaly, Volos, Greece

1. Introduction

Obstructive Sleep Apnea Syndrome (OSAS) is a common sleep-related breathing disorder affecting 5% of the general population (Young et al., 2002). OSAS is characterized by periodic complete or partial cessation of breathing while sleeping. These recurrent events of breathing result in fragmented sleep and recurrent hypoxemia (reductions in hemoglobin oxygen levels) (American Academy of Sleep Medicine, 1999). It has been documented that OSAS causes excessive daytime sleepiness, mood changes and dysfunctions in several cognitive domains (Engleman & Joffe, 1999; Tsara et al., 2009). However, there are different opinions on which cognitive abilities are affected mostly by OSAS and on the exact nature of cognitive decline. The comparison of the findings of research studies is difficult because of differences in severity of disease, criteria that are used to assess the severity of syndromes and different sample sizes (Quan et al., 2006). Other variables such as the sensitivity of neuropsychological battery chosen (Quan et al., 2006) and different group ages are also confounding factors (Mathieu et al., 2008). Nevertheless, in this chapter an effort is made to review studies which examined neurocognitive deficits in OSAS as well as those which reported the Continuous Positive Pressure Therapy (CPAP) treatment effects on several cognitive domains found to be impaired in OSAS. In addition, the most frequent explanations concerning the mechanism of neurocognitive deficits in OSAS patients and the neuroanatomical pathophysiology of OSAS are discussed.

2. Obstructive sleep apnea – Hypopnea syndrome

Obstructive sleep apnea is part of a spectrum of sleep related breathing disorders which also includes central sleep apnea (CSA) (apnea without respiratory effort, defined as 50% or more of respiratory events are central), mixed sleep apnea (episodes of obstructive sleep apnea and central sleep apnea), upper airway resistance syndrome (increased respiratory effort without apnea or hypopnea) and snoring (Avidan, 2005; Lim et al., 2007). Obstructive sleep apnea/hypopnea syndrome is defined as an obstruction of airflow for 10 seconds or longer. It occurs when the muscles relax during sleep, causing soft tissue in the back of the throat to collapse and block the upper airway. Apnea is characterized by the cessation of airflow (decrements in airflow of ≥90%) for 10 seconds or more (Avidan, 2005; Lim et al., 2007; Qureshi & Ballard, 2003). On the other hand, hypopnea is usually characterized by a reduction of ≥50% in airflow for 10 seconds associated with a ≥4% decrease in oxygen saturation and/or arousal (Tsai et al., 1999) while in accordance with the American Academy of Sleep Medicine guidelines hypopnea is defined as a decrease of ≥30% in airflow followed by ≥4% oxygen desaturation (Qureshi & Ballard, 2003).

The diagnosis of the syndrome is based on daytime and nocturnal symptoms and especially on a full-night polysomnogram (Andreou et al., 2002), which includes electroencephalographic, electro-oculographic, electromyographic, oxygen saturation, oral and nasal airflow, respiratory effort, electrocardiographic and leg movement recordings (Qureshi & Ballard, 2003). OSAS severity is defined according to apnea-hypopnea index (AHI), by calculating the sum of apneas plus hypopneas per hour of sleep. According to apnea/hypopnea index (AHI), OSAS patients are divided into 3 groups of severity: mild OSAS (AHI≥5), moderate OSAS (AHI= 15-30), and severe OSAS (AHI≥30) (Qureshi & Ballard, 2003; Tsara et al., 2009). The occurrence of OSAS among children is 1-3 % (Beebe & Gozal, 2002). It affects 2% of women and 4% of men in middle age adults (Young et al., 1993). In older adults (≥65 years), it has been reported that 62% of them present hypopnea episodes and 24% have apnea episodes above normative index (Ancoli - Israel et al., 1991). A newest study on a population - based sample of subjects aged 30 to 70 year found that 19% of men and 15% of women have AHI≥ 10 (Durán et al., 2001).

Obstructive sleep apnea syndrome is characterized by a perturbation of the pharyngeal dilator muscles associated with or without faulty upper airway anatomy such as macroglossia, hypertrophy of tonsils and long uvula (Avidan, 2005; Quereshi & Ballard, 2003). Other risks factors that enhance the probability of OSAS are obesity, increased neck circumference, positive family history, male postmenopausal status, Down syndrome, Pierre-Robin syndrome, alcohol consumption before bedtime, tobacco and hypnotics use as well as sleeping in supine position (Qureshi & Ballard, 2003; Sánchez et al., 2009). These factors result in episodes of complete or partial upper airway obstruction during sleep and in increased sleep arousals that terminate the apneic episodes. These disturbing events while sleeping cause decreased oxygen saturation as well as sleep fragmentation (Avidan, 2005, Beebe & Gozal, 2002; Quereshi & Ballard, 2003).

In addition, it has been shown that sleep architecture changes in OSAS (Avidan, 2005; Sanchez et al., 2009). A normal sleep cycle consists of a cycling from non-REM sleep (non-rapid eye movement), which consists of four stages (stage 1, stage 2, stage 3, stage 4), into REM sleep (rapid eye movement) with a periodicity that lasts for about 90 min. As the night goes on, stages 3 and 4 become shorter and REM sleep longer. On the other hand, in OSAS, it has been found that stage 2 is increased and stage 1, stage 3, stage 4 and REM sleep decreased (Avidan, 2005; Sánchez et al., 2009), although there are different opinions on the decreased total time of REM sleep (Kiralti et al., 2010; Yaouhi et al., 2009). This abnormal sleep architecture makes sleep lighter and less restorative (Sánchez et al., 2009).

The most well known symptom of obstructive sleep apnea/hypopnea syndrome is excessive daytime sleepiness (Lim et al., 2007; Ferini-Strambi, 2003), although some studies failed to report daytime somnolence (Barbé et al., 2001; Black, 2003). Daytime sleepiness is usually assessed with Epworth Sleepiness Scale (ESS) (Tsara et al., 2009) and the majority of patients with OSAS report that they fall asleep in quiet and monotonous situations such as watching television, reading a book, or driving a vehicle (Sánchez et al., 2009). Fatigue, non - refreshing sleep, insomnia, loud snoring, gasping, choking, and reports of breathing interruptions by bed partner are common daytime and nocturnal symptoms of sleep apnea (Saunamäki & Jehkonen, 2007). Poor quality of life, poor interpersonal relationships, low work and school efficiency have been observed in OSAS patients (Engleman & Joffe, 1999; Kales et al., 1985). Moreover, patients with OSAS have a high frequency of psychopathology such as depression and hypochondriasis (Kales et al., 1985; Muñoz et al., 2000). In addition, patients with OSAS present increased morbidity due to high rates of cardiovascular diseases and hypertension (Kales et al., 1985; Lattimore et al., 2003) as well as increased mortality (Engleman & Joffe, 1999; Kales et al., 1985).

The treatment of OSAS is based on restoring the upper airway flow. For that reason, the most effective treatment for patients with craniofacial abnormalities is surgical treatment. In the rest of OSAS patients the most effective treatment is the Continuous Positive Pressure Therapy (CPAP) which consists of an air pressure generating device and a fitting mask that is applied over the nose or the mouth of the patient. The positive air pressure maintains upper airway patency and prevents upper airway obstruction while the patients are asleep (Avidan, 2005; Qureshi & Ballard, 2003). CPAP therapy has been shown to improve nocturnal breathing, oxygen saturation (Avidan, 2005), and mean blood pressure (Jaimchariyatam et al., 2010). As a result, it decreases hypertension and the risk of cardiovascular and cerebrovascular events (Lattimore et al., 2003). CPAP therapy also decreases daytime sleepiness (Muňoz et al., 2000) and improves OSAS patients' mood (Engleman et al., 1994) and quality of life (Engleman et al., 1999). However, these positive effects have not been always reported (Barbé et al., 2001).

3. Neurocognitive deficits in obstructive sleep apnea syndrome

Patients with OSAS show deficits across a wide range of cognitive functions including attention, memory, psychomotor speed and visuospatial abilities, constructional abilities, executive functions and language abilities (Andreou & Agapitou, 2007; Engleman & Joffe, 1999; Findley et al., 1986).

3.1 Attention

Patients with obstructive sleep apnea syndrome have been found to show a decline in vigilance (Aloia et al., 2004; Beebe et al., 2003; Décary et al., 2000; Rouleau et al., 2002) and in complex attention (Lau et al., 2010), such as sustained attention (Kotterba et al., 1998), and selective attention (Kotterba et al., 1998). More specifically, research has shown that severe OSAS patients are characterized by diffused impairments in vigilance (Findley et al., 1986; Lim et al., 2007; Muñoz et al., 2000,) and in sustaining attention and alertness (Findley et al., 1986; Lim et al., 2007). It has been shown that a group of OSAS patients of similar severity of disease, displayed poor performance in Stroop Color, TR2 (Reaction Time Test) (Ferini-Strambi et al., 2003), digit symbol and Steer Clear test (Kingshott et al., 2000), tests which assess selective attention, sustained attention and vigilance. The study of Mathieu et al. (2008) is consistent with these results and shows that a group of 28 patients with severe OSAS and mild hypoxemia, compared to 30 controls, gave low scores in sustaining attention and vigilance measured with four-choice reaction time test.

Moderate and severe OSAS patients have been found to show diffused impairment in vigilance assessed with the Steer-Clear test (Engleman et al., 1994). Moreover, a large majority of moderate and severe sleep apnea patients demonstrated attention deficits on vigilance, selective, sustained and divided attention (Mazza et al., 2005). On the other hand, there have been studies on moderate and severe OSAS patients that failed to report deficits in attention measured with digit symbol test (Pierobon et al., 2008), digit span, and letter-sequence subtasks of Wechsler test (Yaouhi et al., 2009).

Moderate OSAS patients performed normally in digit symbol, digit forward subtest of WAIS, Paced Auditory Serial Addition Test (PASAT), and Steer clear tests that assess sustained, divided attention and vigilance (Monasterio et al., 2001). Twigg et al. (2010) did not observe significant attention deficit assessed with Stroop Color test, digit span forward and Trail Making Test A (TMT A) in mild-to-severe OSAS patients. Mild and moderate OSAS patients, compared to a healthy control group, did not present any significant impairments in attention either (Quan et al., 2006). Finally, there has not been observed any poor performance on Steer Clear test and Trail Making test A in patients with mild OSAS (Engleman et al., 1999). In conclusion, there is not any significant attention decline in non - homogenous groups of patients and only severe OSAS patients present poor performance in attention tasks.

3.2 Psychomotor speed

Several studies (Décary et al., 2000; Lau et al., 2010; Rouleau et al., 2002) have noted decrements in psychomotor efficiency, which appeared to be the most consistent explanation for characterizing the profile of neuropsychological test results among OSAS patients. Lim et al. (2007) compared normative data to severe OSAS patients' performance in psychomotor tasks and found a decline in psychomotor speed measured with Digit symbol, Digit vigilance, Trail Making Test A and Stroop color test. However, differences among severe OSAS patients and healthy controls in Trail making test performance have not been always detected (Mathieu et al., 2008). There has been some evidence for psychomotor speed deficit in moderate and severe OSAS patients (Felver - Gant et al., 2007). Yaouhi et al. (2009) also observed a decreased performance in Purdue Pegboard test in a similar group of patients compared to healthy controls. In a recent study, Twigg et al., (2010) did not observe any psychomotor deficits in mild-to-severe OSAS patients measured with TMT. Finally, patients with mild and moderate OSAS compared to controls did not show any significant poor performances on Grooved Pegboard test (GPT), digit symbol or digit search tasks (Quan et al., 2006). Therefore, it is concluded that attention decline prevalence is higher in severe OSAS patients than in moderate or mild OSAS patients.

3.3 Memory and learning

There is a significant number of studies which have shown a serious decline in memory and learning abilities in OSAS patients (Décary et al., 2000), such as episodic memory (Daurat et al., 2008), short-term memory (Borak et al., 1996; Findley et al., 1986; Naëgelé et al., 1998), long-term verbal memory (Aloia et al., 2003) and verbal and visual learning abilities (Feuerstein et al., 1997). In contrast to studies that did not show any immediate memory decline in severe OSAS patients (Grenèche et al., 2011; Mathieu et al., 2008), other studies found that OSAS patients' performance was poor in short-term verbal memory tests such as digit span test and word list recall (Borak et al., 1996; Lee et al., 2009). The study of Lim et al. (2007) compared normative data to severe OSAS patients' performance on Hopkins Verbal Learning Test (HVLT) and showed a diffused impairment in verbal short and long-term learning and memory. Another study showed that 50% of their OSAS patients presented poor performance in Wechsler memory scale, whereas only 9% of their patients had difficulties in both short and long-term memory (Kales et al., 1985). However, a short-term and long-term verbal memory decline was not always found in severe OSAS patients with an average AHI of 54,95 per hour (Ferini-Strambi et al., 2003). Patients with severe OSAS compared with healthy controls, preserved a good short-term memory and long-term episodic memory measured with digit span forward, immediate recall of Rey Auditory Verbal Learning Test (RAVLT), Digit span backward and delayed recall of RAVLT task. Procedural memory measured with Mirror tracing test was also found intact. Only the performance in immediate recall and the learning of story B of Wechsler memory scale was found decreased (Mathieu et al., 2008).

Regarding working memory, some studies did not find a significant decline in patients with severe OSAS (Ferini-Strambi et al., 2003; Mathieu et al., 2008), whereas other studies did (Grenèche et al., 2011). Severe OSAS patients' also present visual (Borak et al., 1996; Lee et al., 2009; Ferini - Strambi et al., 2003) and spatial memory decline (Borak et al., 1996). Moderate and severe OSAS patients have been presented with poor verbal immediate and delayed recall measured with HVLT (Felver - Gant et al., 2007) RAVLT and Logical Memory Test (Findley et al., 1986; Torreli et al, 2011). However, no significant deficits in episodic memory, measured with verbal logical memory and visual memory of Wechsler test have been observed by Yaouhi et al. (2009). Interestingly, only paired associates - learning curve and percent of retained items in family pictures was impaired (Yaouhi et al., 2009). Pierobon et al. (2008) found significantly lower scores on short-term memory (digit span), and on spatial short-term memory tests (Corsi block test) in their OSAS patients sample in contrast to long-term verbal memory (prose memory test) which was intact. Working memory problems have also been found in moderate and severe OSAS patients assessed with 2-back working memory test, Paced Auditory Serial Addition Test (PASAT) (Felver -Gant et al., 2007) and digit span backward (Torreli et al., 2011). In contrast to this, Yaouhi et al. (2009) did not find any working memory problems in a group of patients of similar severity. No differences between normal and mild-to-severe patients in visual memory and verbal working memory have been found by Twigg et al. (2010). Only immediate and delayed recall of logical memory test as well as spatial working memory were impaired (Twigg et al., 2010). Finally, patients with moderate OSAS did not show any decline in visual or verbal memory assessed with Wechsler Memory Scale (WMS) (Monasterio et al., 2001). Therefore, it seems that memory decline is equivocal in non severe patients and in groups of patients that were not homogenous in OSAS severity.

3.4 Visuospatial and motor constructional abilities

Patients with severe OSAS have been found to have poor visuospatial and constructional abilities measured with tests such as Rey-Ostrerrieth and Purdue Pegboard (Ferini - Strambi et al., 2003). Aloia et al. (2003) also found poor constructional abilities in severe OSAS patients measured with visual motor integration (VMI) test. Moderate and severe OSAS patients scored lower on Rey-Ostrerrieth copy task in comparison to copy drawings and Rey-Ostrerrieth figure recall (Torelli et al., 2011).

3.5 Executive abilities

The majority of the studies have found executive dysfunctions related to mental flexibility, planning, working memory, analysis, synthesis and organizational skills in OSAS patients (Lau et al., 2010; Saunamäki & Jehkonen, 2007). Low scores in tests such as TMT, block design, Intra-Extra Dimensional Set Shifting test (Meurice et al., 1996; Saunamäki et al., 2009), verbal fluency (Andreou & Agapitou, 2007), digit symbol and copying the Rey - Osterrieth complex figure have been observed in many studies (Feuerstein et al., 1997; Naëgelé et al., 1998). Executive dysfunctions, measured with Raven matrices, Digit symbol, phonemic task of verbal fluency, Letter-number sequencing, Stroop Color-Word test and TMT B, have been observed in patients with severe OSAS (Aloia et al., 2003; Bardwell et al., 2001; Lim et al., 2007; Ferini - Strambi et al., 2003). On the other hand, Mathieu et al. (2008) failed to find several noteworthy low scores in trail making B and Wisconsin test.

Regarding moderate and severe OSAS patients, it has been found that they performed poorly in Trail making test B (Engleman et al., 1994; Felver - Gant et al., 2007) in Stroop test and Digit span (Torelli et al., 2011). On the other hand, there are studies on moderate and severe OSAS patients that did not report any impairment in executive functions assessed with TMT (Pierobon et al., 2008), the phonological task of verbal fluency and Raven matrices (Torelli et al., 2011; Yaouhi et al., 2009).

Mild-to-severe OSAS patients have been documented to have significant impairments in mental shift, planning and working memory measured with Stroop test, Raven matrices, digit span backward and trail making test, and had a minimal decline in phonemic fluency (Twigg et al., 2010). In mild and moderate OSAS patients, Quan et al. (2006) found that executive functions, as measured with Stroop test and Trail making B, were affected a little. In addition, moderate OSAS patients were found to perform among the typical range in digit symbol, block design, PASAT and verbal fluency test (Engleman et al., 1999; Monasterio et al., 2001). Regarding patients' performance on TMT, Monasterio et al. (2001) observed a significant decline in contrast to the findings of Engleman et al. (1999) who did not demonstrate this decline.

It is remarkable that some researchers have found that patients' performance on TMT B (Naëgelé et al., 1998; Ferini –Strambi et al., 2003), Wisconsin card sorting test (Salorio et al., 2002) and letter verbal fluency (Naëgelé et al., 1998; Torelli et al., 2011) are normal although their performance was poor in the rest of neuropsychological tests that are sensitive to the detection of executive dysfunctions. One possible explanation is that there is a pattern of both intact and impaired cognitive functions in OSAS patients that make the executive impairments difficult to detect (Lis et al., 2008). More specifically, Grenèche et al. (2011) proposed that there is a specific working memory deficit associated with complex memory tasks and high level memory scanning. Additionally, it has been suggested that deficits in tasks that require high executive functions are apparent only over the course of the day due to circadian variations or duration of time spent awake (Lis et al., 2008).

3.6 Language functions

Most studies on OSAS patients focus more on cognitive functions such as attention, memory and executive functioning rather than on language abilities. Probably, this is associated with the fact that attention and memory problems are more easily noticed by patients, their bed partners and doctors, than language deficits. It has been reported that 62% of OSAS patients show speech disorders, which correlate with sleep deprivation and its effects on neuromotor function (Monoson & Fox, 1987). Furthermore, there have been reports on OSAS patients that have shown significant semantic language deficits (Andreou & Agapitou, 2007; Feuerstein et al., 1997; Lee et al., 2009), although this has not always been found (Beebe et al., 2003). More specifically, Lim et al. (2007) compared normative data to severe OSAS patients' performance in a verbal fluency test and found a significant impairment in semantic language in 30,4 % of this patient group. Other researchers also noted low scores in verbal fluency tests (Aloia et al., 2003; Bardwell et al. 2001). On the other hand, Ferini - Strambi et al. (2003) have failed to show any significant decline in language abilities concerning semantic verbal fluency in OSAS patients while on the other hand their phonemic verbal fluency was found to be impaired (Ferini - Strambi et al., 2003).

Moderate and severe OSAS patients have been found to show similar performance on semantic word fluency compared to healthy controls (Torelli et al., 2011). Minimal differences between mild -to- severe OSAS patients and healthy volunteers on semantic and phonemic verbal fluency are documented by Twigg et al. (2010). Moderate OSAS patients' verbal fluency was also found to be within normal range by Monasterio et al. (2001). An interesting finding is that mild and moderate OSAS adolescents have shown significantly lower scores on semantic and phonemic tasks of verbal fluency. It is suggested that OSAS occurrence during critical ages of brain growth and development such as childhood and adolescence may cause notable language decline (Andreou & Agapitou, 2007).

4. Neurocognitive improvement on OSAS patients after CPAP treatment

Recent studies have shown that CPAP treatment is related to specific cognitive improvements (Avidan, 2005; Naëgelé et al., 1998). Sánchez et al. (2009), in a clinical review, have concluded that CPAP is effective in reducing symptoms of sleepiness, and improves some cognitive functions. Studying cognitive improvement after CPAP therapy is essential to draw safe results about the permanent cognitive dysfunctions owing to OSAS effects.

4.1 Attention

It has been found that a 1-week CPAP treatment improved attentional ability, although the effect was not significantly beneficial for the patients (Bardwell et al., 2001). Studies that have determined the effects of a 2-week CPAP treatment on severe OSAS patients found a significant improvement in vigilance, alertness and sustained attention (Ferini - Strambi et al., 2003; Lim et al., 2007). Research studies that assessed attention after 4 weeks of CPAP treatment also confirmed this improvement in vigilance and attention (Aloia et al., 2001; Engleman et al., 1994). Engleman et al. (1999) found that a 4-week CPAP treatment had a significant positive impact on attentional abilities measured with PASAT test and digit symbol test. However, this group of patients with mild OSAS did not show a significant improvement on Steer Clear test. Patients using CPAP for more than 12 weeks showed an even greater improvement in vigilance than patients who were on a 4-week CPAP treatment (Aloia et al., 2001). Another study that evaluated the effects of 3-month CPAP treatment on severe OSAS patients, found an improvement in vigilance and sustained attention performances, assessed with Conner's continuous performance test (Aloia et al., 2003). Studies that evaluated alertness, vigilance and sustained attention after 6 and 12 months CPAP treatment also found a significant decrease in these cognitive dysfunctions (Kingshott, et al., 2000; Kotterba et al., 1998; Muñoz et al., 2000).

On the other hand, Engleman et al. (1998), in a small sample of 23 OSAS patients who were on a 4-week CPAP treatment, did not observe any improvement in attention measured with PASAT test, SteerClear test, TMT and digit symbol test. Barbé et al. (2001) found that a 6-week CPAP treatment in 55 non sleepy patients with severe OSAS did not modify the patients' performance in vigilance and attention, measured with PASAT, TMT and digit symbols. Pelletier-Fleury et al. (2004) also failed to find any significant improvement in attention measured with TMT in patients who were on a 6-month CPAP treatment. However, in this study, OSAS patients were not equaled in terms of age.

4.2 Psychomotor speed

Bardwell et al. (2001) showed that a 1-week CPAP treatment did not improve very severe OSAS patients' performance in Stroop Test and TMT. On the other hand, Lim et al. (2007) have shown that a 2-week CPAP treatment can significantly decrease the time to complete tests that measure psychomotor speed, such as digit vigilance, Stroop test and Trail Making Test A in severe OSAS patients. Studies on the effects of 3- and 6-month CPAP therapy on cognitive functions of severe OSAS patients observed a decrease in motor speed functions assessed with Purdue Pegboard test (Aloia et al., 2003) and in reaction time measured with TMT, PASAT test (Hoy et al., 1999) and digit symbol test (Kingshott et al., 2000). However, psychomotor speed improvement was not always found in moderate and severe OSAS patients (Felver - Gant et al., 2007) and non sleepy patients (Barbé et al., 2001). In another study, Engleman et al. (1998) did not find psychomotor speed improvement on severe OSAS patients after 4 weeks CPAP treatment. Finally, another study assessing the long-term effects of CPAP, (Muñoz et al., 2000) found that a 1-year CPAP therapy changed only a little OSAS patients' reaction time measured with Psychometer vigilance test.

4.3 Memory and learning

Short-term CPAP treatment for 1 or 2 weeks did not notably improve severe OSAS patients' short- after and long–term verbal memory, visuospatial and working memory, as well as learning ability measured with Hopkins verbal learning test, digit span and Brief visuospatial memory test (Bardwell et al., 2001; Lim et al., 2007). On the other hand, Ferini - Strambi et al. (2003), found that 2-weeks and 4-months CPAP therapy had a significant positive impact on visuospatial learning tasks on 23 severe OSAS patients. According to other studies, a 3-month CPAP treatment had a positive effect on non-verbal recall task (Aloia et al., 2003) and working memory task (Felver - Gant et al., 2007). Borak et al. (1996) found that 20 severe OSAS patients who were on a 3-month CPAP treatment had a significant improvement in recent verbal, visual and spatial memory. In addition, an over 12-month CPAP therapy resulted in considerable improvement on verbal, visual and spatial memory in severe OSAS patients (Borak et al., 1996).

On the other hand, a 1.5-months of CPAP treatment did not modify memory functions of non sleepy patients with severe OSAS (Barbé et al., 2001). Short-term memory impairment was also persistent in OSAS patients despite 4 and 6 months CPAP treatment (Feuerstein et al., 1997; Naëgelé et al., 1998) in contrast to learning disabilities and long-term memory decline (Feuerstein et al., 1997) which improved.

4.4 Visuospatial and motor constructional abilities

It has been observed that severe OSAS patients' performance in assembly trail of Purdue Pegboard test improved significantly after 2-weeks (Ferini - Strambi et al., 2003), 3-months (Aloia et al., 2003) and 4-months CPAP treatment (Ferini - Strambi et al., 2003). However, no significant improvement in tasks that require high mental processes such as visual motor integration (VMI) was observed (Aloia et al., 2003). No significant improvement has been found in Rey - Osterrieth complex figure after 4-months (Ferini - Strambi et al., 2003) and 6 months CPAP therapy (Saunamäki et al., 2009). The above findings led Aloia et al. (2004) to conclude that CPAP treatment failed to improve patients' performance in constructional tasks.

4.5 Executive abilities

Short-term CPAP treatment for 1 and 2 weeks did not improve significantly patients' performance in Stroop Color - Word test, TMT B and Letter - number sequencing (Bardwell et al., 2001; Lim et al, 2007). However, 3-week and 4-week CPAP treatment has been shown to improve mental flexibility measured with TMT (Engleman et al., 1994; Meurice et al., 1996). Engleman et al. (1999) observed that patients'performance in digit symbol and PASAT test was improved, in contrast to TMT and blocks design performance (Engleman et al., 1999). Longer CPAP therapy (3-months) has been found to reverse the impairment in executive functions, since patients improved their performance in Verbal fluency test - Phonemic task and Trail making test B (Aloia et al., 2003), in contrast to another research study which did not find this improvement (Felver-Gant et al., 2007). Longer CPAP treatment for 4 or 6 months has also been found to improve executive functions, such as planning capacities and working memory (Feuerstein et al., 1997; Naëgelé et al., 1998; Saunamäki et al., 2009). Yet, patients with 6 months CPAP treatment did not completely reverse executive dysfunctions measured using Rey - Osterrieth complex figure test (Saunamäki et al., 2009). It seems that high order executive functions or specific domains of executive functions do not improve after CPAP treatment.

4.6 Language functions

There are a few research studies that explored the effects of CPAP treatment on language functions. 1- to 2-week treatment with CPAP failed to improve significantly patients' performance in verbal fluency tasks (Bardwell et al., 2001; Lim et al, 2007) and in Boston naming test (Aloia et al., 2003). A study on severe OSAS patients found that their semantic verbal fluency performance improved after a 15-day CPAP treatment although there was not a statistically significant difference between the healthy subjects' performance and that of OSAS patients before the treatment (Ferini - Strambi et al., 2003).

In conclusion, cognitive deficits in OSAS patients are partially reversible if treated with CPAP. More specifically, CPAP seems to improve only some aspects of cognitive functions. Neurocognitive deficits in high executive functions and verbal fluency do not seem to improve after CPAP treatment (Ferini - Strambi et al., 2003; Montplaisir et al., 1992). It is possible that hypoxemia may have caused permanent brain injury. On the other hand, cognitive tasks such as attention, psychomotor speed and memory that require low mental activation seem to improve after CPAP treatment. It is suggested that the improvement of these cognitive functions are due to improvement of daytime sleepiness and quality of sleep. The diversity in research results reflects differences in methodology, treatment duration, low tolerance of treatment, severity of OSAS, insufficiently sensitive neuropsychological measures and variability of the sample (Sánchez et al., 2009).

5. Mechanism of cognitive impairment in OSAS patients

The cause of cognitive deficits in OSAS patients is complicated. Some researchers have shown a significant correlation between cognitive impairment and daytime sleepiness related to sleep fragmentation resulting from frequent apneas (Valencia-Flores et al., 1996; Verstraeten, 2007) while others attribute cognitive decline to nocturnal hypoxemia (Berry et al., 1986; Findley et al., 1986). Finally, some researchers attribute cognitive impairments to a combination of PSG parameters (AHI, sleep arousals, oxygen desaturation, sleep architecture) (Cheshire et al., 1992; Quan et al., 2006).

More specifically, Verstraeten et al. (2004) proposed that low order deficits such as attentional decline and slow mental processing underlie the more complex deficits found in executive functions. In this study, attention, vigilance and executive functions were assessed with TMT A, B, Stroop color -Word test and Symbol digit Modalities. The cognitive decline was comparable to the decline found after sleep loss. It has been concluded that sleep disruption has a pervasive influence on cognitive functions and affects not only underlying lower level processes such as arousal and alertness, but also higher - level cognitive processes such as executive functioning. In other words, high order cognitive dysfunction can be explained by impairment in both attentional decline and psychomotor speed decrements due to sleepiness (Verstraeten & Raymond, 2004). However, a discussion of sleep fragmentation and hypoxemia is limited in this model.

Another explanation for the cognitive deficits found in OSAS patients suggested that attentional deficits and memory impairments are affected by sleep fragmentation while impairments in executive functions, in constructional abilities, in motor tasks and in language are caused by hypoxemia (Bérard et al., 1991; Kotterba et al., 1998; Naëgelé et al., 1995). More specifically, attention decline was linked to vigilance impairment that derives from changes in sleep architecture (Bédard et al., 1991; Montplaisir et al., 1992). Ferini-Strambi et al. (2003) also found that sustained attention was correlated with daytime sleepiness. Regarding the relation between psychomotor speed and hypoxemia, a significant interrelation was found (Bédard et al., 1991; Findley et al., 1986; Kotterba et al., 1998; Grenéche et al., 2011). Quan et al. (2006) observed this interrelation in mild and moderate

OSAS patients. More severe oxygen desaturation was associated with poorer motor performance and lower processing speed whereas stage 1 sleep, sleep arousals and daytime sleepiness were not correlated with these deficits (Quan et al., 2006). Regarding memory dysfunctions, it has been found that vigilance impairment due to sleep changes contribute to memory decline (Bérard et al., 1991; Montplaisir et al., 1992). Recently, studies on sleep architecture (percentage of slow wave sleep and rapid eye movements sleep) have shown that sleep architecture is negatively associated with immediate memory (forward digit span) and low level memory scanning (simple Sternberg) (Grenéche et al., 2011). In addition, Daurat et al. (2008) showed that the best predictor of episodic memory deficit was the number of microarousals. Constructional abilities have been found to positively associate with the time that oxygen saturation levels are below 80% (Aloia et al., 2003). Executive dysfunctions and hypoxemia seem to be interrelated (Findley et al., 1986; Montplaisir et al., 1992). Ferini-Strambi et al. (2003) showed a significant correlation between the time of oxygen saturation (SaO_2) below 90% or lowest peaks of SaO_2 and the phonemic fluency or the Rey figure in severe OSAS patients. It has been reported that working memory and high-speed memory scanning deficits, factors pertaining to executive functions, are associated with the degree of hypoxemia (mean SaO_2) (Aloia et al., 2003; Grenéche et al., 2011). Regarding verbal disabilities, it has been found that hypoxia could predict patients' performance on verbal fluency test (Berry et al., 1986).

However, this explanation of cognitive deficits needs further elucidation as there are studies that failed to associate memory functions with sleep arousals, sleep architecture (Findley et al., 1986), daytime sleepiness (Lojander et al., 1999) or severity of disease (Lojander et al., 1999; Twigg et al., 2010). Some other studies found a link between hypoxia and attention (Kotterba et al., 1998), verbal and non-verbal memory (Berry et al., 1986; Findley et al., 1986) as well as delayed recall (Aloia et al., 2003). On the other hand, the total time of SWS and REM amount were associated with language and executive functions respectively (Lee et al., 2009). Moreover, there is a research study which failed to associate executive functions, such as working memory, with hypoxia (Felver-Gant et al., 2007). Some other studies found that a specific cognitive decline such as verbal delayed memory impairment is associated with both sleep fragmentation and oxygen desaturation (Aloia et al., 2003; Kiralti et al., 2010).

Beebe and Gozal (2002) have suggested that the frontal lobes of the brain are affected by sleep fragmentation and hypoxemia. Sleep fragmentation is proposed to affect frontal lobes by disrupting the normal restorative processes of sleep, while hypoxemia causes cellular changes in the prefrontal cortex. A recent study on a small group of severe OSAS patients suggested that both hypoxia and sleep fragmentation contribute to frontal dysfunction (Xi et al., 2011). However, this explanation model of cognitive deficits includes exclusion of brain regions other than frontal lobe and little discussion of the nuances of executive functions. Moreover, there are studies that do not ascribe cognitive dysfunctions to both hypoxia and sleep deprivation, i.e., in tasks that assess verbal short-term and long-term memory, non verbal memory, constructional abilities, language (Mathieu et al., 2008; Pierobon et al., 2008; Torelli et al., 2011), attention and executive functions (Lis et al., 2008; Mathieu et al., 2008; Mazza et al., 2005).

Another model, the microvascular theory, has been proposed by Aloia et al (2004). This model suggests that a vascular compromise might exist in the small vessels of the brain and the intermittent hypoxemia of OSAS may affect the regions of the brain that are metabolically active during hypoxemia. Microvascular disease of small vessels that feed white matter of the brain may result in deficits of attention, mental processing, memory executive functions, motor speed and coordination. Recent studies have shown that hypercapnia, cortical and sympathetic activation in OSAS patients cause cardiovascular, cerebrovascular and metabolic disease as well as sudden death (Lloberes et al., 2011). More specifically, repetitive episodes of deoxygenation and reoxygenation increase the production of proinflammatory cytokines (TNF), C-reactive protein and chemoreceptors that are associated with the development of atherosclerosis and high arterial pressure (Lloberes et al., 2011). However, hypoxia, hypercapnia, sleep fragmentation, hemoglobin levels, inflammation parameters and comorbidities are unlikely to account for all cognitive dysfunctions (Dodd et al., 2010).

Beebe (2005) proposed that multiple factors affect the neurocognitive functions in OSAS. It has been suggested that sleep fragmentation and hypoxemia effects are intermingled and synergistic. He proposed that these synergistic mechanisms interact with vulnerable brain regions such as hippocampus, prefrontal cortex, subcortical gray and white matter, suggesting the potential involvement of small vessels in the brain. Regarding the complexity of higher order cognitive abilities such as executive functions, Beebe (2005) suggested that these higher order functions may be dependent on task demands, or the environment of testing, while some specific deficits may be related to some tasks but not others. Other factors such as sociodemographic factors, previous experience on testing and genetic endowment, may also affect cognitive performance (Beebe, 2005). Moreover, Mathieu et al. (2008) found that younger OSAS patients are more sensitive than older OSAS patients to sleep defragmentation and hypoxia. Another study found that socioeconomic status and adolescent cognitive ability may explain verbal disability, verbal memory decline, or rate of impairment in memory (Richards et al., 2005). Finally, Alchanatis et al. (2005) have proposed that intelligence and cognitive functions are interrelated. In other words, high - intelligence may have a protective effect against cognitive decline in OSAS patients, due to increased cognitive reserve.

6. Neuroanatomical pathophysiology of OSAS

In obstructive sleep apnea syndrome, compared to other sleep disorders, at least two primary nocturnal abnormalities occur: hypoxemia and sleep fragmentation. It has been found that a decreased oxygen transport to brain cells modifies ion channels (potassium, sodium, calcium) and as a result cell excitability increases. In addition, it causes alterations in neurotransmitters (dopamine, acetylcholine, ATP), and reduces respiration followed by enhancement of sympathetic and respiratory activities which result in changes involving modification in signaling pathways, in neuromodulators and their receptors as well as genome effects (Areza-Fegyveres et al., 2010; Powell, 2007). It has also been found that frequent oxygen desaturation during everyday activity elevates choline level in frontal brain areas and high levels of choline damage myelin and membrane precursors (Gibson et al., 1981). Hypoxia is also associated with enhancement of hemoglobin concentration level, which can affect cognitive abilities (Grant et al., 1982). Moreover, it may increase hematocrit level and angiogenesis through enhancement of production of vascular growth factors (Areza-Fegyveres et al., 2010). Finally, it is believed that hypoxia, inflammation and oxidative stress initiate the process of endothelian dysfunction that plays a significant role in vascular tone and cellular growth (Butt et al., 2010). Some regions of the brain, such as the hippocampus, basal ganglia, cerebellum, occipital cortex and frontal regions are more susceptible to oxygen deprivation than others (Martin et al., 2011). More specifically, functional magnetic resonance image (fMRI) studies revealed a significant gray matter loss and atrophy in several brain regions including cortex, hippocampus and striatum suggesting that chronic exposure to hypoxia results in neuronal damage and impaired cognitive functions (Maiti et al., 2008; Shukitt-Hale et al., 1996).

Regarding sleep loss effects on brain, it has been found that it decreases pineal melatonin production which causes disturbances in circadian physiology of cells, organs, neurochemicals, neuroprotective and other metabolic functions (Jan et al., 2010). Moreover, it have been found that short-term and long-term sleep deprivation has both been associated with the upregulation of hundreds of genes in the cerebral cortex and other brain areas. This includes genes that are associated with energy metabolism, memory formation, memory consolidation, protein synthesis and synaptic depression (Cirelli et al., 2006). It is well established that chronic sleep deprivation or sleep fragmentation in healthy subjects may cause decline in alertness, simple attention, psychomotor speed as well as learning, memory, working memory and executive functions (Killgore, 2010; Whitney & Hinson, 2010; Reynolds & Banks, 2010). A functional magnetic resonance imaging (fMRI) study has shown the negative impact of sleep deprivation on specific brain regions, such as temporal to parietal regions and frontal lobe regions (Jan et al., 2010). In addition, it has been suggested that long-term sleep deprivation may cause permanent neuronal alterations especially in memory related brain regions, such as hippocampus (Jan et al., 2010). Killgore (2010) observed that chronic sleep deprivation is followed by reduced activation of frontal and parietal networks and alters functioning within the thalamus.

Regarding the neuropathophysiology of OSAS, patients are presented with blood flow reduction during apneic episodes in left frontal and temporal lobes (Kiralti et al., 2010). Yaouhi et al. (2009) found a right-lateralized decreased brain metabolism in precuneus, middle and posterior cingulated gyrus, and the parieto - occipital cortex, as well as the prefrontal cortex (Yaouhi et al., 2009). Joo et al. (2007) also found reduced cerebral blood flow during wakefulness in bilateral hippocampal gyri, right lingual gyrus, precentral gyrus, and cuneus in patients with severe OSAS. These findings may partly explain the deficit in memory, spatial learning, executive function, and attention which are frequently found in OSAS patients (Joo et al., 2007). Xi et al. (2011), using fMRI, observed that OSAS patients showed a decreased mismatch-related activation in frontal regions such as prefrontal cortex and anterior cingulate, whereas an increased activation was only found in the right anterior prefrontal gyrus. Another study (Joo et al., 2009) which used fMRI to assess gray matter volume in OSAS patients, has found reduced brain gray matter concentration in left gyrus rectus, bilateral superior frontal gyri, left precentral gyrus, bilateral frontomarginal gyri, bilateral anterior cingulated gyri, right insular gyrus, bilateral caudate nuclei, bilateral thalami, bilateral amygdalo hippocampi, bilateral inferior temporal gyri and bilateral quadrangular and biventer lobules in cerebellum. These results suggest that memory impairment, executive dysfunctions, cardiovascular disturbances, and dysregulation of autonomic and respiratory control might be related to morphological differences in the brain gray matter areas (Joo et al., 2009). Yaouhi et al. (2009) observed gray matter loss in frontal and temporo-pareieteo-occipital cortices, the thalamus, hippocampal region, some basal ganglia and cerebellar regions mainly in the right hemisphere. Brain morphological changes have also been found in moderate and severe OSAS patients. Volumes of cortical gray matter, such as right and left hippocampus and more lateral temporal areas were also found to be smaller in severe OSAS patients compared to controls (Torelli et al., 2011).

As we have seen, hypoxia and sleep fragmentation cause cellular and molecular changes that lead to disruption of functional homeostasis and altered neuronal and glial viability within particular brain regions (Beebe & Gozal, 2002; Morrell et al., 2003), such as frontal lobe (Beebe et al., 2002 Fuster, 2000; Koechlin et al., 1999) and temporal cortex (Yaouhi et al., 2009). Moreover, hypoxia and sleep deprivation modulate the expression of inflammatory mediators such as interleukins and tumor necrosis factor alpha (Butt et al., 2010). In summary, the pathophysiology of cognitive deficits in OSAS patients is multifactorial. Since OSAS affect multiple brain regions, brain damages may result from several etiologies such as hypoxemia, sleep deprivation, small vessel damages, chronic inflammation, all of which can result in local ischemic episodes (Matthews & Aloia, 2011).

7. Conclusions

In this thorough review of literature, we have shown that the majority of OSAS patients suffer from attentional, memory and psychomotor speed decline, while others present impairments in high order cognitive functions such as executive and language functions. CPAP treatment is not always helpful in improving cognitive functions, suggesting that OSAS may cause permanent damages in specific brain regions. The effects of sleep fragmentation, hypoxemia, low CBF, inflammation parameters and vascocerebral diseases on cognitive functions are intermingled and synergistic. However, these conclusions need to be treated with caution since most studies are not homogeneous in OSAS severity. Moreover, the diversity in the findings of the research studies presented may be due to differences in methodology and in the types of neuropsychological tests which were used to assess cognitive functions. Furthermore, the treatment duration, low tolerance of treatment, and disease duration are not often taken into account in most studies. Therefore, more research is needed to elucidate the etiology of OSAS and investigate further to what extent sleep architecture, cerebral blood flow, gas blood, inflammation parameters, co-morbidities or even socioeconomic factors have a negative impact on cognitive functions in OSAS patients.

8. References

Alchanatis, M., Zias, N., Deligiorgis, N., Amfilochiou, A., Dionellis, G. & Orphanidou, D. (2005). Sleep apnea-related cognitive deficits and intelligence: an implication of cognitive reserve theory. *Journal of Sleep Research*, Vol. 14, No.1, (March 2005), pp. 69-75, ISSN 0962-1105

Aloia, M.S., Arnedt, J.T., Davis, J.D., Riggs, R.L. & Byrd, D. (2004). Neuropsychological squealae of obstructive sleep apnea-hypopnea syndrome: a critical review. *Journal of the International Neuropsychological Society*, Vol. 10, No. 5, (September 2004), pp. 772-785, ISNN 1355-6177

Aloia, M.S., Di Dio, L., Ilniczky, N., Perlis, M.L., Greenblatt, D.W. & Giles, D.E. (2001). Improving compliance with nasal CPAP and vigilance in older adults with OAHS. *Sleep Breathing*, Vol. 5, No. 1, (February 2002), pp. 13-21, ISSN 1520-9512

Aloia, M.S., Ilniczky, N., Di Dio, P., Perlis, M.L., Greenblatt, D.W. & Giles, D.E. (2003). Neuropsychological changes and treatment compliance in older adults with sleep apnea. *Journal of Psychosomatic Research*, Vol. 54, No. 1, (January 2003), pp. 71-76, ISSN 0022-3999

American Academy of Sleep Medicine Task Force. (1999). Sleep-related breathing disorders in adults: recommendations for syndrome definition and measurement techniques in clinical research. *Sleep*, Vol. 22, No. 5, (August 1999), pp.667-689, ISSN 0161-8105

Ancoli - Israel, S., Kripke, D.F., Klauber, M.R., Mason, W.J., Fell, R. & Kaplan, O. (1991). Sleep-Disordered Breathing in Community-Dwelling Elderly. *Sleep*, Vol. 14, No. 6, (December 1991), pp. 486–495, ISSN 0161-8105

Andreou. G. & Agapitou, P. (2007). Reduced language abilities in adolescents who snore. *Archives of Clinical Neuropsychology*, Vol. 22, No. 2, (February 2007), pp. 225 - 9, ISSN 0887-6177

Andreou, G., Galanopoulou, G., Gourgoulianis, A., Karapetsas, A. & Molyvas, P. (2002). Cognitive status in Down syndrome individuals with sleep disordered breathing deficits (SDB). *Brain and Cognition*, Vol. 50, No. 1, (October 2002), pp. 145 -149, ISSN 0278-2626

Areza - Fegyveres, R., Kairalla, R.A., Carvalho, C.R.R. & Nitrini, R. (2010). Cognition and chronic hypoxia in pulmonary diseases. *Dementia & Neuropsychologia*, Vol. 4, No. 1, (March 2010), pp. 14-22, ISSN 1980 - 5764

Avidan, A.Y. (2005). Sleep disordered breathing in the geriatric patient population. *Advances in Cell Aging and Gerontology*, Vol. 17, No. 1, (April 2005), pp. 79-112, ISSN 1566-3124

Barbé, F., Mayoralas, L.R., Duran, J., Masa, J.F., Maimó, A., Montserrat, J.M., Monasterio, C., Bosch, M., Ladaria, A., Rubio, M., Rubio, R., Medinas, M., Hernandez, L., Vidal, S., Douglas, N.J. & Agusti, A.G.N. (2001). Treatment with continuous positive pressure in not effective in patients with sleep apnea but no daytime sleepiness. A randomized, controlled trial. *Annals of Internal Medicine*, Vol. 134, No. 11, (June 2001), pp. 1015-1023, ISSN 0003-4819

Bardwell, W.A., Ancoli-Israel, S., Berry, C.C. & Dimsdale, J.E. (2001). Neuropsychological effects of one-week continuous positive airway pressure treatment in patients with obstructive sleep apnea: a placebo-controlled study. *Psychosomatic Medicine*, Vol. 63, No. 4, (August 2001), pp. 579–584, ISSN 0033-3174

Beebe, D. W. (2005). Neurobehavioral effects of obstructive sleep apnea: An overview and heuristic model. *Current Opinion in Pulmonary Medicine*, 11, 494–500.

Beebe, D.W. & Gozal, D. (2002). Obstructive sleep apnea and the prefrontal cortex: towards a comprehensive model linking nocturnal upper airway obstruction to daytime cognitive and behavioral deficits. *Journal Sleep Research*, Vol. 11, No. 6, (November 2005), pp. 1-16, ISSN 1070-5287

Beebe, D.W., Groesz, L., Wells, C., Nichols, A. & McGee, K. (2003). The neuropsychological effects of obstructive sleep apnea: a meta-analysis of norm-referenced and case-controlled data. *Sleep*, Vol. 26, No. 3, (May 2003) pp. 298-307, ISSN 0161-8105

Bérard, M.A., Montplaisir, J., Richer, F., Rouleau, I. & Malo, J. (1991). Obstructive sleep apnea syndrome: pathogenesis of neuropsychological deficits. *Journal of Clinical and Experimental Neuropsychology*, Vol. 13, No. 6, (November 1991), pp. 950- 964, ISSN 1380-3395

Berry, D.T., Webb, W.B., Block, A.J., Bauer, R.M., Switzer & D.A. (1986). Nocturnal hypoxia and neuropsychological variables. *Journal of Clinical and Experimental Neuropsychology*, Vol. 8, No. 3, (June 1986), pp. 229-38, ISSN 1380-3395

Black, J. (2003). Sleepiness and residual sleepiness in adults with obstructive sleep apnea. *Respiratory Physiology & Neurobiology*, Vol. 36, No. 2-3, (July 2003), pp. 211-220, ISSN 1569-9048

Borak, J., Cieslicki, J.K., Koziej, M., Matuszewski, A. & Zielinski, J. (1996). Effects of CPAP treatment on psychological status in patients with severe obstructive sleep apnoea. *Journal of Sleep Research*, Vol. 5, No. 2, (June 1996), pp. 123-127, ISSN 0962-1105

Butt, M., Dwivedi, G., Khair, O. & Lip, G.Y.H. (2010). Obstructive sleep apnea and cardiovascular disease. *International Journal of Cardiology*, Vol. 139, No. 1, (February 2010), pp. 7-16, ISSN 1874-1754

Cheshire, K., Engleman, H., Deary, I., Shapiro, C. & Douglas, N.J. (1992). Factors impairing daytime performance in patients with sleep apnea/hypoapnea syndrome. *Archives of Internal Medicine*, Vol. 152, No. 2, (March 1992), pp. 538–541, ISSN 0003-9926

Cirelli, C. (2006). Cellular consequences of sleep deprivation in the Brain. *Sleep Medicine Reviews*, Vol. 10, No. (October 2006), pp. 307–321, ISSN 1087-0792

Daurat, A., Foret, J., Bret-Dibat, J.L., Fureix, C. & Tiberge, M. (2008). Spatial and temporal memories are affected by sleep fragmentation in obstructive sleep apnea syndrome. *Journal of Clinical and Experimental Neuropsychology*, Vol. 30, No. 1, (January 2008), pp. 91-101, ISSN 1744-411X

Décary, A., Rouleau, I. & Montplaisir, J. (2000). Cognitive deficits associated with sleep apnea syndrome: a proposed neuropsychological test battery. *Sleep*, Vol. 23, No.3, (May 2000), pp. 369-381, ISSN 0161-8105

Dodd, J.W., Getov, S.V. & Jones, P.W. (2010). Cognitive function in COPD. *The European Respiratory Journal*, Vol, 35, No. 4, (April 2010), pp. 913-22, ISSN 1399-3003

Durán, J., Esnaola, S., Rubio, R. & Iztueta, A. (2001). Obstructive sleep apnea - hypopnea and related clinical features in a population-based sample of subjects aged 30 to 70 yr. *American Journal of Respiratory and Critical Care Medicine*, Vol.163, No.3, (March 2001), pp. 685-689, ISSN 1073-449X

Engleman, H. & Joffe, D. (1999). Neuropsychological function in obstructive sleep apnoea. *Sleep Medicine*, Vol. 3, No. 1, (March 1999), pp. 59-78, ISSN 1087-0792

Engleman, H.M., Kingshott, R.N., Wraith, P.K. & Mackay, T.W. (1999). Randomized Placebo-controlled Crossover Trial of Continuous Positive airway Pressure for Mild Sleep Apnea/Hypopnea syndrome. *American Journal of Respiratory and Critical Care Medicine*, Vol. 159, No. 2, (February 1999), pp. 461-467, ISSN 1073-449X

Engleman, H.M., Martin, S.E., Deary, I.J. & Douglas, N.J. (1994). Effect of continuous positive airway pressure treatment on daytime function in sleep apnoea / hypopnoea syndrome. *Lancet*, Vol. 343, No. 8897, (March 1994), pp. 572-575, ISSN 0140-6736

Engleman, H.M., Martin, S.E., Kingshott, R.N. & Mackay, T.W. (1998). Randomised placebo controlled trial of daytime function after continuous positive airway pressure

(CPAP) thereapy fro the sleep apnoea/hypopnea syndrome. *Thorax*, Vol. 53, No. 5, (May 1998), pp. 341 - 345, ISSN 0040-6376

Felver-Gant, J.C., Bruce, A.S., Zimmerman, M., Sweet, L.H., Milmman, R.P. & Aloia, M.S. (2007). Working memory in obstructive sleep apnea: construct validity and treatment affects. *Journal of Clinical Sleep Medicine*, Vol. 3, No. 6, (October 2007), pp. 589-594, ISSN 1550-9389

Ferini - Strambi, L., Baietto, C., Gioia, M.R., Castaldi, P., Castronovo, C., Zucconi, M. & Cappa, S.F. (2003). Cognitive dysfunction in patients with obstructive sleep apnea (OSA): partial reversibility after continuous positive airway pressure (cpap). *Brain Research Bulletin*, Vol. 61, No. 1, (June 2003), pp. 87-92, ISSN 0361-9230

Feuerstein, C., Naëgelé, B., Pepin, J.L. & Levy, P. (1997). Frontal lobe-related cognitive functions in patients with sleep apnea syndrome before and after treatment. *Acta Neurologica Belgica*, Vol. 97, No. 2, (June 1997), pp. 96-107, ISSN 0300-9009

Findley, L.J., Barth, J.T., Powers, D.C., Wilhoit, S.C., Boyd, D.G. & Suratt, P.M. (1986). Cognitive impairment in patients with obstructive sleep apnea and associated hypoxemia. *Chest*, Vol. 90, No. 5., (November 1986), pp. 686-690, ISSN 0012-3692

Fuster, J.M. (2000). Prefrontal neurons in networks of executive memory. *Brain Research Bulletin*, Vol. 52, No. 5, (July 2000), pp. 331-336, ISSN 0361-9230

Gibson, G.E., Pulsinelli, W., Blass, J.P. & Duffy, T.E. (1981). Brain dysfunction in mild to moderate hypoxia. *American Journal of Medicine*, Vol. 70, No. 6, (June 1982), pp. 1247 - 1254, ISSN 0002-9343

Grant, I., Heaton, R.K., McSweeny, A.J., Adams, K.M. & Timms, R.M. (1982). Neuropsychologic findings in hypoxemic chronic obstructive pulmonary disease. *Archives of Internal Medicine*, Vol. 142, No. 8, (August 1982), pp. 1470-6, ISSN 0003-9926

Grenèche, J., Krieger, J., Bertrand, F., Erhardt, C., Maumy, M. & Tassi, P. (2011). Short-term mempry performances during sustained wakefulness in patients with obstructive sleep apnea-hypopnea syndrome. *Brain and Cognition*, Vol. 75, No. 1, (February 2011), pp. 39-50, ISSN 1090-2147

Hoy, C.J., Vennelle, M., Kingshott, R.N. & Engleman, H.M. (1999). Can intensive support imrove continuous positive airway pressure use in patients with sleep apnea/hypopnea syndrome?. *American Journal of Respiratory and Critical Care Medicine*, Vol. 159, No. 4 Pt 1, (April 1999), pp. 1096 - 1100, ISSN 1073-449X

Jaimchariyatam, N., Rodriguez, C.L. & Budur, K. (2010). Does CPAP treatment in mild obstructive sleep apnea affect blood pressure?. *Sleep Medicine*, Vol. 11, No. 9, (October 2011), pp. 837-842, ISSN 1878-5506

Jan J.E., Reiter, R.J., Bax, M.C.O., Ribary U., Freeman, R.D. & Wasdell, M.B. (2010). Long-term sleep disturbances in children: A cause of neuronal loss. *European Journal of Pediatric Neurology*, Vol. 14, No. 5, (September 2010), pp. 380-390, ISSN 1532-2130

Joo, E.Y., Tae, W.S.,Han, S.J., Cho, Jae-Wook. & Hong, S.B.(2007). Reduced cerebral blood flow during wakefulness in obstructive sleep apnea - hypopnea syndrome. *Sleep*, Vol. 30, No. 11, (November 2007), pp. 1515 - 1520, ISSN 0161-8105

Joo, E.Y., Tae, W.S., Lee, M.J., Kang, J.W., Park, H.S., Lee, J.Y., Suh, M. & Hong, S.B. (2009). Reduced brain gray matter concentration in patients with obstructive sleep apnea syndrome. *Sleep*, Vol.33, No. 2, (February 2009), pp.235- 241, ISSN 0161-8105

Kales, A., Caldwell, A., Cadieux, R., Vela-Bueno, A., Ruch, L. & Mayes, S. (1985). Severe obstructive sleep apnea - II: associated psychopathology and psychosocial consequences. *Journal of Chronic Diseases*, Vol. 38, No. 5, (January 1985), pp. 427-434, ISSN 0021-9681

Killgore, W.D.S. (2010). Effects of sleep deprivation on cognition. *Progress in Brain Research*, Vol. 185, No. 1, (November 2010), pp. 105-129, ISSN 1875-7855

Kingshott, R.N., Vennelle, M., Hoy, C.J. & Engleman, H.M. (2000). Predictors of improvements in daytime function outcomes with CPAP therapy. *American Journal of Respiratory and Critical Care Medicine*, Vol. 161, No. 3 Pt 1, (March 2000), pp.866-871, ISSN 1073-449X

Kiralti, P.O., Demir, A.U., Volkan- Salanci, B., Demir, B. & Sahin, A. (2010). Cerebral blood flow and cognitive function in obstructive sleep apnea syndrome. *Hellenic Journal of Nuclear Medicine*, Vol. 13, No. 2, (May - August 2010), pp. 138-143, ISSN 1790-5427

Koechlin, E., Basso, G., Pietrini, P., Panzer, S. & Grafman, J. (1999). The role of the anterior prefrontal cortex in human cognition. *Nature*, Vol. 399, No. 6732, (May 1999), pp. 148–151, ISSN 0028-0836

Kotterba, S., Rasche, K., Widdig, W., Duscha, C., Blombach, S., Schultze-Werninghaus, G. & Malin, J.P. (1998). Neuropsychological investigations and event-related potentials in obstructive sleep apnea syndrome before and during CPAP-therapy. *Journal of the Neurological Sciences*, Vol. 159, No.1, (July 1998), pp. 45-50, ISSN 0022-510X

Lattimore, J., Celermajer, D.S. & Wilcox, I. (2003).Obstructive Sleep Apnea and Cardiovascular Disease. *Journal of the American College of Cardiology*, Vo. 41, No. 9, (May 2003), pp. 1429 -37, ISSN 0735-1097

Lau, E.Y., Eskes, G.A., Morrison, D.L., Rajda, M. & Spurr, K.F. (2010). Executive function in patients with obstructive sleep apnea treated with continuous positive airway pressure. *Journal of International Psychological Society*, Vol. 16, No. 6, (November 2010), pp. 1077-1088, ISSN 1469-7661

Lee, J., Kim, S., Lee, D. & Woo, J. (2009). Language function related to sleep quality and sleep apnea in the elderly. *Sleep Medicine*, Vol. 10, No. 2, (December 2009), pp. s50, ISSN 0

Lim, W., Bardwell, W., Loredo, J., Kim, E., Ancoli-Israel, S., Morgan, E., Heaton, R. & Dimsdale, J. (2007). Neuropsychological Effects of 2-Week Continuous Positive Airway Pressure Treatment and Supplemental Oxygen in Patients with Obstructive Sleep Apnea: A Randomized Placebo-Controlled Study. *Journal of Clinical Sleep Medicine*, Vol. 3, No. 4, (June 2007), pp. 380 - 386, ISSN 1550-9389

Lis, S., Krieger, S., Hennig, D., Roder, C., Kirsch, P., Seeger, W., Gallhofer, B. & Schulz, R. (2008). Executive functions and cognitive subprocesses in patients with obstructive sleep apnoea. *Journal of Sleep Research*, Vol. 17, No. 3, (May 2008), pp. 271–280, ISSN 1365-2869

Lloberes, P., Durán - Cantolla, J., Martinez-Garcia, M.A., Marin, J.M., Ferrer, A., Corral, J., Masa, J.F., Parra, O., Alonso-Alvarez, M.L. & Teran-Santos, J. (2011). Diagnosis and treatment of sleep apnea-hypopnea syndrome. *Archivos de Bronconeumologia*, Vol. 47, No. 3, (March 2011), pp. 143- 156, ISSN 1579-2129

Lojander, J., Kajaste, S., Maasilta, P. & Partinen, M. (1999). Cognitive function and treatment of obstructive sleep apnea syndrome. *Journal of Sleep Research*, Vol. 8, No. 1, (March 1999), pp. 71-76, ISSN 0962-1105

Maiti, P., Singh, S.B., Mallick, B., Muthuraju, S. & Ilavazhagan, G. (2008). High altitude memory impairment is due to neuronal apoptosis in hippocampus, cortex and striatum. *Journal of Chemical Neuroanatomy*, Vol. 36, No. 3-4, (December 2008), pp. 227 - 238, ISSN 0891-0618

Martin, S.E., Bradley, J.M., Buick, J.B., Crossan, A. & Stuartelborn, J. (2011). The effect of hypoxia on cognitive performance in patients with chronic obstructive pulmonary disease. *Respiratory Physiology & Neurobiology*, Vol. 177, No. 1, (June 2011), pp. 46 - 40, ISSN 1878-1519

Mathieu, A., Mazza, S., Decary, A., Massicotte-Marquez, J., Petit, D., Gosselin, N., Malo, J. & Montplaisir, J. (2008). Effects of obstructive sleep apnea on cognitive function: A comparison between younger and older OSAS patients. *Sleep Medicine*, Vol. 9, No. 2, (January 2008), pp. 112-120, ISSN 1389-9457

Matthhews, E.E. & Aloia, M.S. (2011). Cognitive recovery following positive airway pressure (PAP) in sleep apnea. *Progress in Brain Research*, Vol. 190, (May 2011), pp. 71- 88, ISSN 1875-7855

Mazza, S., Pépin, J.L., Naëgelé, B., Plante, J., Deschaux, C. & Lévy, P. (2005). Most obstructive sleep apnoea patients exhibit vigilance and attention deficits on an extended battery of tests. *The European Respiratory Journal*, Vol. 25, No.1, (January 2005), pp. 75-80, ISSN 0903-1936

Meurice, J.C., Marc, I. & Series, F. (1996). Efficacy of auto-CPAP in the treatment of obstructive sleep apnea/hypopnea syndrome. *American Journal of Respiratory and Critical Care Medicine*, Vol. 153, No. 2, (February 1996), pp. 794-798, ISSN 1073-449X

Monasterio, C., Vidal, S., Duran, J., Ferrer, M., Carmona, C., Barbé, F., Mayos, M., Gonzalez-Mangado, N., Montserrat, J., Navarro, A., Barreira, R., Capote, F., Mayaoralas, L.R., Peces-Barba, G., Alonso, J. & Montserrat, J.M. (2001). Effectiveness of continuous positive airway pressure in mild sleep apnea-hypopnea syndrome. *American Journal of Respiratory and Critical Care Medicine*, Vol. 164, No.6, (September 2001), pp. 939-943, ISSN 1073-449X

Monoson, P.K. & Fox, A.W. (1987). Preliminary observation of speech disorder in obstructive and mixed sleep apnea. *Chest*, Vol. 92, No. 4, (October 1987), pp. 670 - 675, ISSN 0012-3692

Montplaisir, J., Bedard, M.A., Richer, F. & Rouleau, I. (1992). Neurobehavioral manifestations in obstructive sleep apnea syndrome before and after treatment with continuous positive airway pressure. *Sleep*, Vol. 15, No. 6, (December 1992), pp. S17-S19, ISSN 0161-8105

Morrell, M.J., McRobbie, D.W., Quest, R.A., Cummin, A.R.C., Ghiassi, R. & Corfield, D.R. (2003). Changes in brain morphology associated with obstructive sleep apnea. *Sleep Medicine*, Vol. 4, No. 5, (September 2003), pp. 451–454, ISSN 1389-9457

Muñoz, A., Mayoralas L.R., Barbé, F., Pericas, J. & Agustí, A.G.N. (2000). Long-term effects of CPAP on daytime functioning in patients with sleep apnoea syndrome. *The European Respiratory Journal*, Vol. 15, No.4, (April 2000), pp. 676- 681, ISSN 0903-1936

Naëgelé, B., Pepin, J.L., Levy, P., Bonnet, C., Pellat, J. & Feuerstein, C. (1998). Cognitive executive dysfunction in patients with obstructive sleep apnea syndrome (OSAS) after CPAP treatment. *Sleep*, Vol. 21, No. 4, (June 1998), pp. 392–397, ISSN 0161-8105

Naëgelé, B., Thouvard,V., Pépin, J.L., Lévy, P., Bonnet, C., Perret, J.E., Pellat,J. & C. Feuerstein, C. (1995). Deficits of cognitive executive function in patients with sleep apnea syndrome. *Sleep*, Vol. 18, No. 1, (January 1995), pp. 43–52, ISSN 0161-8105

Pelletier-Fluery, N., Meslier, N., Gagnadoux, F., Person, C., Rakotonanahary, D., Ouksel, H., Fleury, B. & Racineux, J-L. (2004). Economic arguments for the immediate management of moderate-to-severe obstructive sleep apnoea syndrome. *The European Respiratory Journal*, Vol. 23, No. 1, (January 2004), pp.53-60, ISSN 0903-1936

Pierobon, A., Giardini, A., Fanfulla, F., Callegari, S. & Majani, G. (2008). A multidimensional assessment of obese patients with obstructive sleep apnoea syndrome (OSAS): A study of psychological, neuropsychological and clinical ralationships in a disabling multifaceted disease. *Sleep Medicine*, Vol. 9, No. 8, (December 2008), pp. 882-889, ISSN 1389-9457

Powell, F.L. (2007). The influence of chronic hypoxia upon chemoreception. *Respiratory Physiology & Neurobiology*, Vol. 157, No.1, (July 2007), pp. 154–161, ISSN 1569-9048

Quan, S. F., Wright, R., Baldwin, C.M., Kaemingk, K.L., Goodwin, J.L., Kuo, T.F., Kaszniak, A., Boland, L.L., Caccappolo, E. & Bootzin, R.R. (2006). Obstructive sleep apnea-hypopnea and neurocognitive functioning in the sleep heart health study. *Sleep Medicine*, Vol. 7, No.6, (September 2006), pp. 498-507, ISSN 1389-9457

Qureshi, A. & Ballard, R.D. (2003). Obstructive sleep apnea. The *Journal of Allergy and Clinical Immunology*, Vol. 112, No. 4, (October 2003), pp. 643-51, ISSN 0091-6749

Reynolds, A.C. & Banks, S. (2010). Total sleep deprivation, chronic sleep restriction and sleep disruption. *Progress in Brain Research*, Vol. 185, (November 2010), pp. 91-103, ISSN 1875-7855

Richards, M., Strachan, D., Hardy, R., Kuh, D. & Wadsworth, M. (2005). Lung Function and Cognitive Ability in a Longitudinal Birth Cohort Study, *Psychosomatic Medicine*, Vol. 67, No. 4, (July - August 2005), pp. 602–608, ISSN 1534-7796

Rouleau, I., Décary, A., Chicoine, A.J. & Montplaisir, J. (2002). Procedural skill learning in obstructive sleep apnea syndrome. *Sleep*, Vol. 25, No. 4, (June 2002), pp. 401-411, ISSN 0161-8105

Salorio C.F., White, D.A., Piccirillo, J., Duntley, S.P. & Uhles, M.L. (2002). Learning, memory, and executive control in individuals with obstructive sleep apnea syndrome. *Journal of Clinical and Experimental Neuropsychology*, Vol. 24, No. 1, (February 2002), pp. 93-100, ISSN 1380-3395

Sánchez, A.I., Martínez, P., Miró, E., Bardwell, W.A. & Buela-Casal, G. (2009). CPAP and behavioral therapies in patients with obstructive sleep apnea: Effects on daytime sleepiness, mood, and cognitive function. *Sleep Medicine Reviews*, Vol. 13, No. 3, (June 2009), pp. 223-233, ISSN 1532-2955

Saunamäki, T. & Jehkonen, M. (2007). A review of executive functions in sleep apnea syndrome. *Acta Neurologica Scanvinavica*, Vol. 115, No. 1, (January 2007), pp. 1-11, ISSN 0001-6314

Saunamäki, T., Jehkonen, M., Huupponen, E., Polo, O. & Himanen, S.L. (2009). Visual dysfynction and computational sleep depth changes in obstructive sleep apnea syndrome. *Clinical EEG and Neuroscience*, Vol. 40, No. 3, (July 2009), pp. 162-167, ISSN 1550-0594

Shukitt-Hale, B., Kadar, T., Marlowe, B.E., Stillman, M.J., Galli, R.L., Levy, A., Devine, J.A. & Lieberman, H.R. (1996). Morphological alteration in the hippocampus following hypobaric hypoxia. *Human and Experimental Toxicology*, Vol. 15, No. 4, (April 1996), pp. 312–319, ISSN 0960-3271

Torelli, F., Moscufo, N., Garreffa, G., Placidi, F., Romigi, A., Zannino, S., Bozzali, M., Fasano, F., Giulietti, G., Djonlagic, I., Malhotra, A., Marciani, M. & Guttmann, C. (2011). Cognitive profile and brain morphological changes in obstructive sleep apnea. *NeuroImage*, Vol. 54, No. 2, (January 2011), pp. 787 - 793, ISSN 1095-9572

Tsai, W.H., Flemons, W.W., Whitelaw, W.A. & Remmersa, J.E. (1999). Comparison of apnea-hypopnea indices derived from different definitions of hypopnea. *American Journal of Respiratory and Critical Care Medicine*, Vol. 159, No.1, (January 1999), pp. 43–48, ISSN 1073-449X

Tsara, V., Kaimakamis, E., Serasli, E., Katsarou, Z. & Christaki, P. (2009). Health related of life in Greek patients with sleep apnea-hypopnea syndrome treated with continuous positive airway pressure. *Sleep Medicine*, Vol. 10, No. 2, (February 2009), pp. 217-225, ISSN 1389-9457

Twigg, G.L., Papaioannou, I., Jackson, M., Ghiassi, R., Shaikh, Z., Jaye, J., Graham, K.S. , Simonds, A.K. & Morrell, M.J.(2010). Obstructive Sleep Apnea Syndrome Is Associated with Deficits in Verbal but Not Visual Memory. *American Journal of Respiratory and Critical Care Medicine*, Vol. 182, No.1, (July 2010), pp. 98-103, ISSN 1535-4970

Valencia-Flores, M., Bliwise, D., Guilleminault, C., Cilveti, R. & Clerk, A. (1996). Cognitive function in patient with sleep apnea after acute nocturnal nasal continuous positive airway pressure (CPAP) treatment: sleepiness and hypoxemia effects. *Journal of Clinical and Experimental Neuropsychology*, Vol. 18, No. 2, (April 1996), pp. 197–210, ISSN 1380-3395

Verstraeten, E. (2007). Neurocognitive effects of obstructive sleep apnea syndrome. *Current Neurology and Neuroscience Reports*, Vol. 7, No. 2, (March 2007), pp. 161-6, ISSN 1528-4042

Verstraeten, E., & Cluydts, R., Pevernagie, D. & Hoffmann, G. (2004). Executive function in sleep apnea: Controlling for attentional capacity in assessing executive attention. *Sleep*, Vol. 27, No.4, (June 2004), pp. 685-693, ISSN 0161-8105

Verstraeten, E. & Raymond, C. (2004). Executive control of attention in sleep apnea patients: theoretical concepts and methodological considerations. *Sleep Medicine*, Vol. 8, No. 4, (August 2004), pp. 257 - 267, ISSN 1087-0792

Whitney, P. & Hinson J.M. (2010). Measurement of cognition in studies of sleep deprivation. *Progress in Brain Research*, Vol. 185, (November 2010), pp.37-48, ISSN 1875-7855

Xi, Z., Lin, M., Shunwei, L., Yuping, W. & Luning, W. (2011). A functional MRI evaluation of frontal dysfunction in patients with severe obstructive sleep apnea. *Sleep Medicine*, Vol. 12, No. 4, (April 2011), pp.335-340, ISSN 1878-5506

Yaouhi, K., Bertran, F., Clochon, P., Mezenge, F., Denise, P., Foret, J., Eustache, F. & Desgranges, B. (2009). A combined neuropsychological and brain imaging study of obstructive sleep apnea. *Journal of Sleep Research*, Vol. 18, No. 1, (March 2009), pp.36–48, ISSN 1365-2869

Young, T., Palta, M., Dempsey, J., Skatrud, J., Weber, S. & Badr, S. (1993). The occurrence of sleep-disorded breathing among middle-aged adults. *New England Journal of Medicine*, Vol. 328, No. 17, (April 1993), pp.1230-1235, ISSN 0028-4793

Young, T., Peppard, P.E. & Gottlieb, D.J. (2002). Epidemiology of obstructive sleep apnea: a population health perspective. *American Journal of Respiratory Critical Care Medicine*, Vol. 165, No. 9, (May 2002), pp. 1217 - 1239, ISSN 1073-449X

6

Cognitive Disturbances in Sneddon and Antiphospholipid Syndromes

M. Rahmani, M. El Alaoui Faris, M. Benabdeljlil and S. Aidi
Department of Neurology A and Neuropsychology
Hôpital des Spécialités, University Mohammed V Souissi, Rabat,
Morocco

1. Introduction

Sneddon's syndrome is a rare disease defined by generalised livedo racemosa of the skin and recurrent stroke. It was first described in a patient in 1960 by Champion and Rook (Champion and Rook, 1960), and five years later Sneddon IB suggested the association of livedo and stroke in six new cases (Sneddon, 1965). Sneddon's syndrome may be differentiated according to the presence or absence of circulating antiphospholipid (aPL) antibodies: aPL-positive Sneddon's syndrome and aPL-negative or seronegative Sneddon's syndrome (Ulukaya et al, 2008). Approximately 40% of Sneddon's syndrome patients have aPL antibodies, raising the question of whether Sneddon's syndrome overlaps with primary antiphospholipid antibody syndrome (APS) and systemic lupus erythromatosis (SLE) (Geschwind et al, 1995). APS or Hughes syndrome is a systemic autoimmune disease consisting of thrombosis (venous and/or arterial) and/or pregnancy failure in association with persistent production of aPL antibodies (aPL): anticardiolipin antibodies (aCL) of immunoglobulin G (IgG) and IgM class, lupus anticoagulant (LA) causing prolongation of activated partial thromboplastin time, and/or B2 glycoprotein I antibodies of IgG and IgM class. Although there are overlapping manifestations between Sneddon's syndrome and APS, namely livedo and recurrent thrombotic events, their relationship remains controversial (Francès et al, 1999). Some authors consider aPL-positive Sneddon's syndrome as a primary APS while others support the idea that aPL antibodies are involved in the pathogenesis of Sneddon's syndrome (Fetoni et al, 2000; Hannon et al, 2010; Kalashnikova et al, 1990; Luvisotto Marinho et al, 2007; Sumi et al, 1999). In this article, we will review the clinical and neuropsychological features of Sneddon's syndrome and APS and focus on the seronegative Sneddon's syndrome although the majority of the published data does not make a distinction between seronegative and aPLpositive Sneddon's syndrome.

2. Sneddon's syndrome

Sneddon's syndrome occurs usually among women in their third decade. Most cases are sporadic, but some rare familial cases have been reported (Pettee et al, 1994; Rebollo et al,1983; Scott et al, 1986). Both autosomal dominant and recessive transmissions were noted (Mascarenhas et al, 2003). Livedo racemosa, introduced for the first time in 1907 by Ehrmann, is characterized by a striking violaceous netlike patterning of the skin similar to the familiar livedo reticularis, from which it differs by its location (more generalized and widespread, non-infiltrated, found not only on the limbs but also on the trunk and/or buttocks), its shape (irregular, broken, circular segments) and its persistence with variation of ambient temperature (Uthman and Khamashta, 2006).

The pathogenesis of Sneddon's syndrome remains unclear and the proposed etiology varies from a hypercoagulate state to a primary inflammatory vasculopathy (De Reuck, 2009). The etiology of Sneddon's syndrome is not completely understood. Skin biopsies often fail to yield diagnostic arterial lesions. Selection of the correct biopsy site (seemingly uninvolved skin at the center of a livedo racemosa area), adequate biopsy size (1 to 2 cm), and serial sections are essential for detection of relevant vascular pathology (Zelger et al, 1992). Sensitivity of these biopsies increased from 27% with one biopsy to 80% with 3 biopsies (Wohlrab et al, 2001). Sepp et al, (1995) studied skin specimens of 18 patients with Sneddon's syndrome, and reported that CD3+, UCHL-1+ (ubiquitin carboxy-terminal hydroxylase L1) and HLA-DR+ cells constituted a significant proportion of the inflammatory infiltrate in the early stages, whereas in later stages, endothelial cells and leukocytes were scarce. These data confirmed the hypothesis that Sneddon's syndrome starts as an inflammatory and possibly immunologically mediated disorder, leading to a migration and proliferation of smooth cells of small arteries, resulting in a partial or complete narrowing of the vessel. Others studies did not find inflammatory abnormalities at skin biopsies (Wohlrab et al, 2001). In few studies, brain biopsies have not shown vasculitic or thrombotic changes (Boortz-Marx et al, 1995; Devuyst et al, 1996; Geschwind et al, 1995). The small number of pathological studies makes it difficult to determine whether Sneddon's syndrome is inherently an inflammatory vasculitic or occlusive thrombotic disease (Hannon et al, 2010).

Diagnosis of Sneddon's syndrome is based on the presence of skin livedo and neurological symptoms related to stroke. Neurological manifestations of Sneddon's syndrome range from motor deficit, aphasia, headache, vertigo and seizures (table 1) (Fetoni et al, 2000; Stockhammer et al, 1993; Tourbah et al, 1997). Intracerebral, subarachnoid and intraventricular hemorrhages have also been reported (Bayrakli et al, 2010; Kraemer et Berlit, 2008; Luvisotto Marinho et al, 2007). Few case reports have described seronegative Sneddon's syndrome (Duval et al, 2009; Hanon et al, 2010; Luvisotto Marinho et al, 2007). To our knowledge, only two series have analyzed both patients suffering from Sneddon's syndrome with and without aPL (Francès et al, 1999; Tourbah et al, 1997). No correlation was noted between severity of neurological outcome and the posivity of aPL (Tourbah et al, 1997). No difference beetwen these two subgroups concerning the mean age at first clinical cerebral event was observed (Francès et al, 1999). Seronegative Sneddon's syndrome seems to have larger fishnet pattern of livedo racemosa, less frequent seizures and slower progression (Francès et al, 1999; Hannon et al, 2010).

Sneddon's syndrome is a progressive condition, and the long-term functional status is usually related to the cumulative burden of repeated ischemic infarcts leading to mental deterioration and dementia. Prognosis of untreated Sneddon's syndrome is poor, and about half of the patients suffer long-term disability (Francès et al, 1999; Tourbah et al, 1997). The differential diagnosis should include other neurological diseases associating cutaneous alterations of vascular origin and stroke. One of these rare entities has been described by Divry and Van Bogaert in 1946 and called diffuse leptomeningeal angiomatosis. Divry Van Bogaert's syndrome (DVB) is characterised by recurrent strokes in young patients especially children, preceded by livedo localized mainly on the face and distal extremities. Skin biopsies show no vasculitis, but an increased number of dermal vessels with smooth muscles fibers disposed around them is seen. Cerebral CT scan and MRI in DVB syndrome can be identical to Sneddon's syndrome. Cerebral angiography showing corticomeningeal angiomatosis with collateral vascular anastomosis and narrow and helicine vessels in the midcerebral arteries confirms the diagnostic of Divry Van Bogaert's disease (Guillot et al, 1994). Dego's disease also known as malignant atrophic papulosis, first described in 1942 by Degos, is an another rare syndrome, very similar to Sneddon's syndrome and characterised by thrombo-occlusive vasculopathy affecting the skin and various internal organs. In the skin, Dego's disease initially manifests with erythematous, pink or red papules. These papules heal to leave scars with pathognomonic, central, porcelain white atrophic centers and a peripheral telangiectatic rim leading to atrophy and ulcers of the skin. In the systemic form, gastrointestinal and central nervous system involvements are the most frequent complications (Jura et al, 1994).

Neurological signs	Stockhammer et al, 1995 17 cases	Tourbah et al, 1997 26 cases	Fetoni et al, 2000 9 cases
Motor deficit	70 %	73%	66%
Aphasia	35%	50%	-
Cognitives disorders	-	27%	11%
Neuro-ophtalmic signs	29%	30%	22%
Sensitives signs	76%	19%	-
Seizures	17%	19%	11%
Headache	82%	38%	-
Vertigo	47%	11%	11%
Pseudo-bulbar syndrome	11%	11%	-

Table 1. Neurological features of Sneddon's syndrome in different series

Limited data are available concerning cognitive dysfunction in Sneddon's syndrome. After several years of evolution, 77% of patients with Sneddon's syndrome exhibit signs of mild cognitive vascular impairment with loss of concentration ability, memory disturbances and/or frontal type of behavioral changes (De Reuck, 2009). To date, only three reports have mentioned a detailed psychometric study showing marked deficits in the tests of memory, concentration, attention, visual perception and visuo-spatial construction (Hannon et al, 2010; Montagné de la Roque and al, 2006; Weissenborn et al., 1996). Cognitive disorders especially impairments in concentration and memory are often observed in Sneddon's syndrome without any history of cerebral stroke (Adair et al, 2001; Maamar et al, 2007; Weissenborn et al, 1996; Wohlrab et al, 2006). Evolution of Sneddon's syndrome includes continued cognitive decline and progression of leukoencephalopathy, causing subcortical vascular dementia in 23% of cases and resulting often in disability to get a correct employment (kalashnikova et al, 1990; Kraemer et al, 2008; Maamar et al, 2007; Rebollo et al, 1983; Stephen et Ferguson, 1982; Stockhammer et al, 1993; Weissenborn et al, 1996). In 2003, Boesch et al, did not find this classical pattern of Sneddon's syndrome in a prospective six year follow up study. Results of their study suggest in contrast a low incidence of territorial stroke and dementia but outline progressive leucencephalopathy. Dementia is caused by the recurrence of ischemic, rarely hemorrhagic stroke and it is preceded in half of cases by a transient ischemic attack. The process that leads to neurological dysfunction seems to be both structurally destructive and functionally impairing with neuronal loss (Liberato and Levy, 2007). Rarely, dementia represents the initial symptom of Sneddon's syndrome (Flöel et al, 2002; Maamar et al, 2007).

In Sneddon's syndrome, stroke affects mainly medium-sized arteries and are seen particularly in the territory of the middle and posterior cerebral artery (Maamar et al, 2007; Stockhammer et al, 1993). Infarct of the vertebral basilar territory was present in 47% of cases among 17 patients described by Stockhammer et al in 1993. Basal ganglia are usually normal (Tourbah et al, 1997). Leucoencephalopathy constitutes a classical MRI finding in the evolution of Sneddon's syndrome, localized usually in the posterior subcortical white matter (Boesch et al, 2003; Tourbah et al, 1997). As reported by Tourbah et al in 1997 and Weissenborn et al in 1996, the extent of cerebral infarcts is significantly correlated with the severity of cognitive disorders. The progressive cognitive impairment in Sneddon's syndrome is also, correlated to the degree of white matter changes and the presence of lacunar infarcts (De Reuck, 2009). Moreover the cognitive dysfunction score is related to the brain atrophy score (Weissenborn et al, 1996) and the degree of physical impairment (Tourbah et al, 1997; Weissenborn et al, 1996). In contrast, the duration of the disease seems to have no influence on the degree of cognitive dysfunction (Weissenborn et al, 1996).

There is no current therapeutic consensus well established in the management of Sneddon's syndrome. In the absence of controlled studies, treatment of Sneddon's syndrome remains empirical. Antiplatelets agents and anti-coagulant treatment are most often used. Corticosteroids, azathioprine and cyclophosphamid were administered by some with little success (Zelger et al, 1993). Few reports noted potential therapeutic options for cognitive disorder in Sneddon's syndrome patients, but generally, theses studies did not demonstrate objective improvements on neuropsychological evaluation. Kume et al (1996) treated a 24-year-old man using cyclophosphamide, prednisolone with improvement of psychiatric symptoms and a decreased anticardiolipin level. However, mental abilities remained subnormal. No objective neuropsychological testing was performed. Flöel et al (2002) also reported a 29-year-old woman with Sneddon's syndrome who continued to decline cognitively when treated with steroids, azathioprine and aspirin. The therapy was switched to aspirin plus clopidogrel and the regimen stabilized cognitive function on neuropsychological tests. One other study confirmed subsequent improvement in subjective and objective memory and emotional status in a 46 years old woman suffering from seronegative Sneddon'syndrome using a treatment with cyclophosphamide during 8 months. Authors have suggested therefore that cyclophosphamide should be considered among first line treatment options for patients with Sneddon's syndrome and cognitive impairment (Hannon et al, 2010).

3. Antiphospholipid antibody syndrome

APS is an autoimmune disorder in which autoantibody production can lead to a hypercoagulable state, pregnancy failure and/or a multitude of other systemic manifestations. APS has previously been divided into primary and secondary forms, these last are associated with other connective tissue diseases, mainly SLE. However, this distinction was abandoned in the new classification (The 2006 Sydney Revised Classification Criteria based on the preliminary international Sapporo 1999) (table 2).

Diagnostic criteria for antiphospholipid syndrome
Clinical criteria
- Vascular thrombosis: one or more episodes of arterial, venous or small vessel thrombosis in any tissue or organ (confirmed by imaging or histopathology) - Recurrent pregnancy loss (1 > 10 weeks' gestation, or 3 < 10 weeks' gestation) or one or more premature births due to pregnancy complications
Laboratory criteria
- Lupus anticoagulant in plasma on two occasions at least 12 weeks apart - Anticardiolipin antibodies of IgG and/or IgM isotype on two occasions at least 12 weeks apart - Anti-b2-GPI antibody of IgG or IgM isotype on two occasions at least 12 weeks apart
Antiphospholipid syndrome is considered to be definitely present when at least one clinical criterion and one laboratory criterion are met. Ig: immunoglobulin; GPI: glycoprotein-I.

Table 2. Diagnostic criteria for APS based on the 2006 Sydney update of the 1999 Sapporo classification (Austin and Cohen, 2010)

In addition to peripheral thrombosis affecting any size of vessels, a variety of clinical manifestations is reported: skin disease, cardiac, pulmonary and renal involvement, haematologic manifestations and wide spectrum of neurological disorders (Mayer et al, 2010). Thrombocytopenia is variably present. Neurological features of APS are dominated by the presence of ischaemic stroke which is the most common neurological manifestation (>50% of CNS complications). Other reported neurological manifestations include cerebral venous thrombosis, migraines, seizures, chorea, transverse myelitis and multiple sclerosis like syndrome (Austin and Cohen, 2010). Two clinical subgroup of APS are now identified. Catastrophic APS is characterized by life-threatening acute multiple organ failure from extensive microvascular thrombosis ('thrombotic storm'). Laboratory evidence of disseminated intravascular coagulation can occur. Suggested precipitants of this syndrome include infection, oral contraceptives, surgery and withdrawal of anticoagulation. The mortality rate is approximately 50%. The second subset is called Seronegative APS which includes patients exhibiting clinical manifestations of APS, without any recognized aPL. Subsequent repeat aPL testing can be positive (Austin and Cohen, 2010).

Several studies suggest an association between aPL and cognitive dysfunction based on microthrombotic events or vasculopathy. The underlying mechanism of cognitive deficits is not clear. Hypothesis of recurrent cerebral ischemia or a direct effect of aPL disrupting neuronal function, like it is shown in experimental studies on animal models has been issued (Katzav et al, 2001).

The majority of studies concerning cognition in APS patients included also cases of SLE with aPL. Although there have been no studies to date that have accurately identified the frequency of neuropsychological manifestations in APS, studies in SLE patients with or without aPL provide excellent models for the analysis of neurocognitive dysfunction (Erkan et al, 2011).

Results of several series indicated that a majority of patients with APS (combined primary and SLE-related APS) had cognitive deficits affecting like in Sneddon's syndrome, mainly memory, concentration, complex attention and verbal fluency (Tektonidou et al, 2006).

Two studies have examined the cognitive function in primary APS patients compared to controls or other patient groups. Jacobson et al (1999) examined neuropsychological functioning in 27 young patients with elevated levels (>10 IU) of aCL IgG. Compared with 27 age and education-matched controls, there were group differences in domain scores of working memory, executive functions, verbal learning, memory and visuospatial functioning. The overall frequency of impaired neuropsychological performance was greater among individuals with aPL than controls (33% versus 4% respectively) suggesting subtle neurological involvement. Tektonidou et al (2006), examined 39 patients with primary APS, 21 patients with SLE-related APS and 60 healthy controls using a neuropsychological battery measuring attention, learning, memory, executive functions and visuospatial skills and depression. Results indicated that 42% of the 60 patients with APS (combined primary and SLE-related APS) had cognitive deficits compared with 18% of healthy controls with deficits most common in complex attention and verbal fluency. There was no difference in cognitive performance between patients with primary APS and those with SLE-associated APS (Erkan et al, 2011). Maeshima et al (1992) analyzed 21 SLE patients with aPL and noted abnormal findings in verbal learning and visuoconstructive skills in 72% of patients. Otherwise, LA positive patients had poor results in verbal memory, attention, cognitive flexibility and psychomotor speed tests in comparison with LA negative patients (Denburg et al, 1997; Leritz et al, 2000; Menon et al, 1999). Positive LA test has been found to be more frequent (15,7%) in SLE patients with cognitive disorder compared to the SLE patients without cognitive impairment (Sanna et al, 2003). Hanley et al (2004) reported also that patients with persistently elevated IgG aCL had a significant decline in psychomotor speed, while those with persistently elevated IgA aCL had decline in conceptual reasoning and executive ability.

Chapman et al (2002) studied 23 patients with primary APS and found that 13 (56%) fulfilled criteria for vascular dementia. Patients with dementia were older, had more CT scan abnormalities and more electroencephalography changes than those without dementia. The "Euro-Phospholipid consortium", did not find the same results in their cohort of 1000 APS patients, only 25 cases (2,5%) had vascular dementia.

Other studies of primary APS or asymptomatic aPLpositive patients have shown that cognitive deficits may be present independent of any history of known central nervous system involvement. These patients may complain of difficulty with memory, attention, and concentration; or the dysfunction may be subclinical and apparent only with neuropsychological testing (Austin and Cohen, 2010; Erkan et al, 2011). Erkan et al,(2010) in a 10-years follow-up study of 66 patients with primary APS, found that 3 patients (<30 years old) developed dementia, independently of the presence of cerebrovascular accidents. In a recent study of 25 patients with APS followed between 1983 and 2003, previous history of stroke and/or transient ischemic stroke was present respectively in only 11 and 2 patients, whereas, silent brain infarcts were present in 14 (47%) patients. Dementia was the presenting manifestation of the APS in 11 (37%) patients (Gomez-Puerta et al, 2005).

Although relatively few studies have been conducted, neuroimaging abnormalities have been reported in primary APS patients presenting with high levels of overt clinical neurological and psychiatric syndromes. Infarcts and hyperintense white matter foci are the most common abnormalities seen on cerebral CT scan or MRI in APS patients. However, most neuroimaging studies reported include patients with both APS and lupus (Erkan et al, 2011).

Cortical and subcortical infarcts are the most frequent findings. Gomez-Puerta et al (2005) studied neuroimaging findings in combined lupus/APS group of 30 patients and reported cortical infarcts in 63% of patients, subcortical infarcts in 30%, basal ganglia infarcts in 23% and signs of cerebral atrophy in 37%. Other ischaemic lesions such as lacunar and periventricular infarcts are not uncommon. Cerebral atrophy and white matter lesions (leukoaraiosis), similar to the lesions found in Binswanger's disease, are often seen, especially in elderly APS patients(Gomez-Puerta et al, 2005). Chapman et al (2002) reported that only half of their demented APS patients had abnormal CT scans and suggested that the demented APS patients with normal CT scans may have micro-lesions. Of those with dementia, six had generalized atrophy and seven of the scans had focal lesions consistent with vascular pathology.

Only one study of primary APS patients has investigated MRI abnormalities and their relation to cognitive dysfunction. Significant correlation between cognitive dysfunction and the presence of white matter lesions was reported in APS patients with and without central nervous system involvement. In 23 APS patients with central nervous system involvement, 12 patients (52%) had white matter lesions with 100% in the periventricular area. Of the 36 APS patients without central nervous system involvement, 8 (22%) of the patients had white matter lesions with 88% in the periventricular location. Cognitive deficits were identified in 7 of those patients. A significant correlation was reported between cognitive deficits and white matter lesions across the two groups (Tektonidou et al, 2006). MRI spectroscopy is a predictive tool when compared to conventional parenchymal MRI in patients with APS, cognitive decline and normal brain MRI. These results corroborate the impression of subclinical neuronal damage induced by disease activity. When multimodal imaging techniques are used assessing not only neurometabolic patterns (MR spectroscopy), but also perfusion (SPECT) and morphological abnormalities (conventional MRI), the predictive power seems to be increased (Liberato and Levy, 2007). Kao et al (1999) studied 22 patients with primary APS with only mild neuropsychiatric manifestations (headache, depression, personality disorders, memory loss and cognitive function deficits) and normal brain MRI. They found that 16 (73%) of the patients had abnormal SPECT findings, mainly diffuse hypoperfusion lesions in cerebral cortex.

Management of APS consists of initial therapy with low molecular weight heparin followed by oral anticoagulation. The duration of therapy depends on any additional risk factors, the location, severity, patient age and the relative risk of further thrombosis versus haemorrhage due to anticoagulation. Several strategies have been suggested for the treatment of dementia in APS patients. The management of atherogenic risk factors (i.e. diabetes, hypertension, hyperlipidaemia) is crucial. However, there is still no evidence that aspirin alone is effective in treating patients with a diagnosis of dementia. Some findings of improvement of cognitive function in the APS patients who underwent anticoagulation therapy have been reported (Hughes et al, 2001). In dementia associated with APS, anticoagulant treatment is recommended. Furthermore, the compliance of demented patients is usually poor, which requires special thought and attention (Gomez-Puerta et al, 2005).

In conclusion, seronegative Sneddon's syndrome should be distinguished from Sneddon's syndrome with aPL which should be considered as a subgroup of APS. Cognitive disorders in both Sneddon' syndrome and APS seem to be similar affecting mainly memory, attention and concentration functions. They represent sometimes the inaugural symptom in a patient without any history of known ischemic stroke. Recurrent stroke may lead to multi-infarct dementia and early retirement in young people. Prognosis depends on early diagnosis. More subtle cognitive dysfunction can be shown. These troubles are related to posterior cortical infarcts or to leucoencephalopathy. Treatment should be aggressive in case of cognitive disturbances in Sneddon's syndrome or APS.

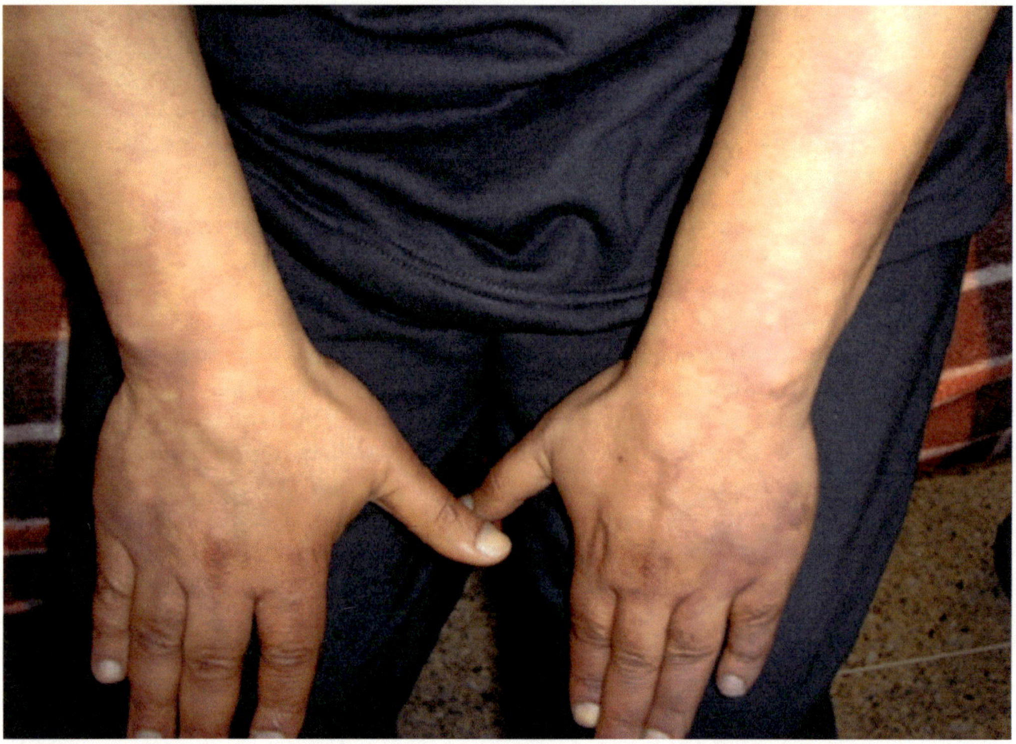

Fig. 1. Livedo racemoca affecting upper limbs in a patient with Sneddon's syndrome (personal figure)

4. References

Adair JC, Digre KB, Swanda RM, Hartshorne MF, Lee RR, Constantino TM, et al. Sneddon syndrome: a cause of cognitive decline in young adults. Neuropsychiatry, Neuropsychology, and Behavioral Neurology (2001);14:197–204.

Austin S and Cohen H. Antiphospholipid syndrome. Medicine (2010); 38,2:101-104.

Bayrakli F, Erkek E, Kurtuncu M, Ozgen S. Intraventricular Hemorrhage as an Unusual Presenting Form of Sneddon Syndrome. World Neurosurg (2010) 73, 4:411-413.

Boesch SM , P Plörer AL, Auer AJ J and al. The natural course of Sneddon's syndrome: clinical and magnetic resonance imaging findings in a prospective six year observation study. J Neurol Neurosurg Psychiatry (2003); 74:5 42-5 44.

Boortz-Marx RL, Clark HB, Taylor S, Wesa KM, Anderson DC. Sneddon's syndrome with granulomatous leptomeningeal infiltration. Stroke (1995);26:492–5.

Champion RH, Rook A. Livedo reticularis.Proc R Soc Med (1960);53:961-962.

Chapman J, Abu-Katash M, Inzelberg R et al. Prevalence and clinical features of dementia associated with the antiphospholipid syndrome and circulating anticoagulants. J Neurol Sci (2002); 203 - 204:81 - 4.

Denburg SD, Carbotte RM, Denburg JA. Psychological aspects of systemic lupus erythematosus: cognitive function, mood, and self-report. J. Rheumatol. 24 (1997) 998–1003.

De Reuck J.L. Sneddon's syndrome. Journal of the Neurological Sciences 283 (2009) 240-320.

Devuyst G, Sindic C, Laterre E. Neuropathological findings of a Sneddon's syndrome presenting with dementia not preceeded by clinical cerebrovascular events. Stroke (1996);27:1008–9.

Duval A, Darnige L, Glowacki F, Copin MC, Martin De Lassalle E, Delaporte E and Eric Auxenfants E. Livedo, dementia, thrombocytopenia, and endotheliitis without antiphospholipid antibodies: Seronegative antiphospholipid-like syndrome. J Am Acad Dermatol, (2009) 61, 6: 1076-1078.

Erkan D, Kozora E, Lockshin MD. Cognitive dysfunction and white matter abnormalities in antiphospholipid syndrome. Pathophysiology 18 (2011) 93–102.

Ehrmann S. Ein Gefaessprozess Bei Lues. Wien Med Wochenschr (1907); 57:777-82.

Fetoni V, Grisoli M M, S Salmaggi A, Carriero R, Girotti F. Clinical and neuroradiological aspects of Sneddon´s syndrome and primary antiphospholipid antibody syndrome: a follow-up study. Neurol S Sci (2000); 21: 157-164.

Flöel A, Imai T, Lohmann H, Bethke F, Sunderkötter C, Droste DW. Therapy of Sneddon's syndrome. Eur Neurol (2002);48: 126- 132.

Francès C, Papo T, Wechsler B, Laporte JL, Biousse V, Piette JC. Sneddon syndrome with or without antiphospholipid antibodies. A comparative study in 46 patients. Medicine (1999);78:209–19.

Geschwind DH, FitzPatrick M, Mischel PS, Cummings JL. Sneddon's syndrome is a thrombotic vasculopathy: neuropathologic and neuroradiologic evidence. Neurology (1995);45:557–60.

Gomez-Puerta JA, Cervera R, Calvo LM, Gomez-Anson B, Espinosa G. Dementia associated with the antiphospholipid syndrome:clinical and radiological characteristics of 30 patients. Rheumatology (Oxford) 44 (2005) 95–99.

Guillot D, Salamand P, Tomasini P, Briant JF, Brosset C. Accidents vasculaires cérébraux ischémiques du sujet jeune et livedo réticulaire. A propos d'un cas de syndrome de Sneddon ou de Divry-Van Bogaert. Annales de Radiologie (1994); 37: 281-5.

Hanly JG, McCurdy G, Fougere L, Douglas J, Thompson K. Neuropsychiatric events in systemic lupus erythematosus: attribution and clinical significance. J Rheumatol (2004); 31:2156–62.

Hannon PM, Kuo SH, Strutt AM, York MK, Kass JS. Improvement of neurological symptoms and memory and emotional status in a case of seronegative Sneddon syndrome with cyclophosphamide. Clinical Neurology and Neurosurgery 112 (2010) 544–547.

Hughes GR, Cuadrado MJ, Khamashta MA, Sanna G. Headache and memory loss: rapid response to heparin in the antiphospholipid syndrome. Lupus (2001);10:778.

Jacobson MW, Rapport LJ, Keenan PA, Coleman RD, Tietjen GE. Neuropsychological deficits associated with antiphospholipid antibodies. J. Clin. Exp. Neuropsychol. (1999) 21: 251–264.

Jura E, Palasik W, Meurer M, Palester-Chlebowczyk M, Czlonkowska A. Sneddon's syndrome (livedo reticularis and cerebrovascular lesions) with antiphospholipid antibodies and severe dementia in a young man: a case report. Acta Neurol Scand (1994), 89: 143-146.

Kalashnikova LA, Nasonov EL, Kushekbaeva AE, Gracheva LA. Anticardiolipin antibodies in Sneddon´s syndrome. Neurology (1990);40(3 Pt 1): 464-467.

Kao CH, Lan JL, Hsieh JF and al. Evaluation of regional cerebral blood flow with 99mTc-HMPAO in primary antiphospholipid antibody syndrome. J Nucl Med (1999);40:1446 - 50.

Katzav A, Pick CG, Korczyn AD, Oest E, Blank M, Shoenfeld Y, Chapman J. Hyperactivity in a mouse model of the antiphospholipid syndrome. Lupus 10 (2001) 496–499.

Kraemer M and Berlit P. Cerebral haemorrhage as the presenting form of Sneddon's syndrome. Clinical Neurology and Neurosurgery (2008) 110 : 532–533.

Kume M, Imai H, Motegi M, Miura AB, Namura I. Sneddon's syndrome (livedo racemosa and cerebral infarction) presenting psychiatric disturbance and shortening of fingers and toes. Internal Medicine (1996);35:668–73.

Leritz E, Brandt J, Minor M, Reis-Jensen F, Petri M. Subcortical cognitive impairment in patients with systemic lupus erythematosus. J.Int. Neuropsychol. Soc. (2000) 6: 821–825.

Liberato B and Levy RA. Antiphospholipid Syndrome and Cognition. Clinic Rev Allerg Immunol (2007) 32:188–191.

Luvisotto Marinho J, Juliato Piovesan E, Pereira Leite Neto M, Kotze LR, De Noronha L, Twardowschy CA, Lange MC, Scola RH, Flumignan Zétola VH, Nóvak EM, Werneck LC. Clinical, neurovascular and neuropathological features in Sneddon's syndrome. Arq Neuropsiquiatr (2007);65(2-B):390-395.

Maamar M, Rahmani M, Aidi S, Benabdeljlil M, El Hassani My R, Jiddane M, Hicham CH, El Alaoui-Faris M. Sneddon's syndrome: study of 15 cases with cerebral arteriography. Rev Neurol (Paris) 2007; 163 : 8-9, 809-816.

Maeshima E, Yamada Y, Yukawa S, Nomoto H. Higher cortical dysfunction, antiphospholipid antibodies, and neuroradiological examinations in systemic lupus Erythematosus. Intern. Med. (1992) 31:1169–1174.

Mascarenhas R, Santo G, Gonçalo M, Ferro Ma,Tellechea O, Figueiredo A. Familial Sneddon's syndrome. Eur J Dermatol (2003); 13: 283–7.

Mayer M, Ceroveca M, Rados M, Cikes N. Antiphospholipid syndrome and central nervous system. Clinical Neurology and Neurosurgery (2010)112: 602–608.

Menon S, Jameson-Shortall E, Newman SP, Hall-Craggs MR, Chinn R, Isenberg DA. A longitudinal study of anticardiolipin antibody levels and cognitive functioning in systemic lupus erythematosus. Arthritis Rheum (1999); 42:735–41.

Montané de la Roque P, Michard JF, Pinganaud-Shrestha C, About I, Campistron E, Malick-Loiseau C, Bories L, Rochet N, Denat S. Dementia revealing a Sneddon's syndrom. Rev Med Interne. (2006); 27(2):162-4. Epub 2005 Nov 10.

Pettee AD, Wasserman BA, Adams NL, McMullen W, Smith HR, Woods SL, Ratnoff OD. Familial Sneddon's syndrome: clinical, hematologic and radiographic findings in two brothers. Neurology (1994); 44: 399-405.

Rebollo M, Val JF, Garijo F, Quintana F, Berciano J. Livedo reticularis and cerebrovascular lesions (Sneddon's Syndrome). Brain (1983), 106: 965-979.

Sanna G, Bertolaccini ML, Cuadrado MJ, Liang H, Khamashta MA. Neuropsychiatric manifestations in systemic lupus erythematosus: prevalence and association with antiphospholipid antibodies. J. Rheumatol. (2003)30: 985–992.

Scott IA, Boyle RS. Sneddon's syndrome. Aust NZ J Med (1986); 16: 799-802.

Sepp N, Zelger B, Schuler G, Romani N, Fritsch P. Sneddon's syndrome-an inflammatory disorder of small arteries followed by smooth muscle proliferation. Immunohistochemical and ultrastructural evidence. Am J Surg Pathol (1995);19:448-53.

Sneddon IB. Cerebrovascular lesions and livedo reticularis. Br J Dermatol (1965);77:180-185.

Stephens WP, Ferguson JT. Livedo reticularis and cerebrovascular disease. Postgrad Med J (1982), 58: 70-73.

Stockhammer G, Felber SR, Zelger B et al. Sneddon´s syndrome: diagnosis by skin biopsy and MRI in 17 patients. Stroke (1993); 24:6 85-690.

Sumi Y, Ozaki Y, Itoh S, Katayama H, Tanaka S. Cerebral blood flow-SPECT in a patient with Sneddon's syndrome. Ann Nucl M Med (1999); 13: 109- 112.

Tektonidou MG, Varsou N, Kotoulas G, Antoniou A, Moutsopoulos HM. Cognitive deficits in patients with antiphospholipid syndrome: association with clinical, laboratory, and brain magnetic resonance imaging findings. Arch. Intern. Med. (2006) 166: 2278–2284.

Tourbah A, Piette JC, Benoît N, Iba-Zizen MT, Lyon-Caen O, Francès C. Clinical, biological and neuroradiological aspects of Sneddon's syndrome: 26 cases. Rev Neurol (Paris). (1997) Nov;153(11):652-8.

Ulukaya S, Makay O, Icoz G, Demir F, Sezer T. Perioperative management of Sneddon syndrome during thyroidectomy. Journal of Clinical Anesthesia (2008) 20, 458–461.

Uthman IW and Khamashta MA. Livedo Racemosa: A Striking Dermatological Sign for the Antiphospholipid Syndrome. The Journal of Rheumatology (2006); 33:12.

Weissenborn K, Rückert N, Ehrenheim C, Schellong S, Goetz C, Lubach D. Neuropsychological deficits in patients with Sneddon's syndrome. J Neurol. (1996); 243(4):357-63.

Wohlrab J, Fischer M, Wolter M, Marsch WC. Diagnostic impact and sensitivity of skin biopsies in Sneddon's syndrome. A report of 15 cases. Br J Dermatol (2001); 145:285-8.

Wohlrab J, Francès C, Sullivan KE. Strange symptoms in Sneddon's syndrome. Clin Immunol. 2006;119(1):13-5. Epub 2005 Nov 28.

Zelger B, Sepp N, Schmid KW, Hintner H, Klein G, Fritsch PO. Life history of cutaneous vascular lesions in Sneddon's syndrome. Hum Pathol (1992); 23:668-75.

7

Cognitive Features of Vascular Dementia

Oh Dae Kwon
Department of Neurology, Daegu Catholic University Medical Center, and School of Medicine, Catholic University of Daegu
South Korea

1. Introduction

A lot of studies have focused on cerebrovascular disease as an independent cause of dementia. In a study with consecutive stroke patients aged sixty and older, 26.3% of patients were demented three months after the stroke (Desmond et al., 2000). Within the demented patients, 57.1% had dementia directly related with stroke and 38.7% had dementia due to the combined effects of stroke and Alzheimer's disease. Considering high prevalence of stroke, the prevalence of vascular dementia should be substantially high. Therefore early accurate diagnosis is crucial to the effective management of patients with vascular dementia. Recognizing a specific pattern of neuropsychological impairment could be a good diagnostic tool of vascular dementia. However, Cognitive features of vascular dementia are not homogenous because of various features, pathophysiology, and location of cerebrovascular diseases. Adopting the cognitive criteria of Alzheimer's disease, which requires early prominent memory impairment, for use in vascular dementia could be erroneous in many cases of vascular dementia. Memory impairment has been an essential component of the operational criteria of dementia such as Diagnostic and Statistical Manual of Mental Disorders, Fourth Edition (DSM-IV) criteria (American Psychiatric Association, 1994) and even in National Institute of Neurological Disorders and Stroke and the Association Internationale pour La Recherche et l'Enseignement en Neuroscienes (NINDS-AIREN) criteria (McKhann G et al., 1994). On the other hand, in the Alzheimer's Disease Diagnostic and Treatment Center (ADDTC) criteria (Chui et al., 1992) they do not require memory impairment as crucial element but need deterioration of intellectual function sufficient to interfere with customary affairs of life. Until now, many reports showed that frontal executive dysfunction is a prominent symptom of vascular dementia as well as less prominent memory impairment (Bowler et al., 1994, Tatemichi et al., 1992). It could be more appropriate omitting memory impairment as an essential component of the criteria of vascular dementia because of various locations of cerebrovascular lesion and of specified functional areas of human brain. In accordance with such ideas, impairment of two or more cognitive domains, not essentially include memory Impairment, was suggested as the diagnostic requirement of vascular dementia (Bowler & Hachinski, 2003). In this chapter we will focus on subcortical mild cognitive impairment and subcortical ischemic vascular dementia because of the relative homogeneity, higher prevalence (Roman et al., 2002; Erkinjuntti et al., 2000), and distinctive clinical features similar to Alzheimer's disease.

2. Cognitive features of each subtypes of vascular cognitive impairment

2.1 Mild cognitive impairment of vascular origin

Mild cognitive impairment refers to a transitional state between normal cognitive state and dementia (Petersen et al., 1999). In general, neurodegenerative dementia like Alzheimer's disease has insidious onset, slowly progressive cognitive deterioration with few or no focal neurological signs. Mild cognitive impairment in Alzheimer's disease, which shows memory impairment without significant impairment of activities of daily living, may precede clinical stages of dementia. On the other hand, vascular dementia may not be a slowly progressive dementia but could be an abrupt onset cognitive decline followed by stroke. It has long been thought that there was no preceding cognitive impairment, like Mild Cognitive Impairment to Alzheimer's disease, before the beginning of vascular dementia. However, more and more reports support the existence of mild cognitive impairment stages of vascular dementia (Frisoni et al., 2002), which shows less memory impairment and severe executive dysfunction (Kim et al., 2011). Both patients with Parkinson disease and mild cognitive impairment (PD-MCI) and patients with subcortical vascular mild cognitive impairment (svMCI) are known to have cognitive dysfunction especially in frontal lobe function (Caviness et al., 2007; Mckinlay et al., 2009; Frisoni et al., 2002) .

Kim et al (2011) compared the cognitive function of PD-MCI and svMCI to differentiate one from the other (Table 1). Twenty-two PD-MCI and 22 svMCI patients were seen in a neurodegenerative disease clinic and 22 normal controls were also recruited. Every participant took brain magnetic resonance imaging which reveals no significant findings in PD-MCI and in normal controls compared with severe ischemic cerebral white matter lesion in svMCI. Mild cognitive impairment was diagnosed according to the criteria of Petersen (1999). All the patients had subjective cognitive complaint and neuropsychological tests showed cognitive decline in one or more domains. However the cognitive deficits did not result in significant functional decline. svMCI should also meet the criteria of Erkinjunti et al (2000) which mandates minor neurological symptoms and diffuse cerebral white matter lesion demonstrated on magnetic resonance imaging. These three groups were matched in terms of age, gender, and education. The Seoul Neuropsychological Screening Battery (SNSB) (Kang & Na, 2003), a standardized neuropsychological battery, was performed in svMCI and PD-MCI subjects. The battery contains tests for attention, language, praxis, four elements of Gerstmann syndrome, visuoconstructive function, verbal and visual memory, and frontal/executive function. Only several important tests among SNSB were performed in controls. svMCI should meet the criteria modified from those of Erkinjuntti (2000).

2.1.1 Frontal executive function

Frontal executive dysfunction was prominent in both MCI groups after analysis of covariance with depression adjustment. The svMCI group performed lower in word fluency and stroop test than the PD-MCI group.

2.1.2 Memory

Both groups showed decreased performance in verbal and visuospatial memory tests. The PD-MCI group performed lower in the verbal recognition test than the svMCI group, which showed lower visuospatial memory

Variables	PD-MCI(n=22)	svMCI(n=22)	NC(n=22)	*F*	LSD
Word Fluency					
Animal	**11.00(2.98)**	**10.82(2.89)**	**14.50(3.91)**	**6.86***	1=2, 1<3, 2<3
Supermarket	**11.09(3.13)**	**10.05(4.45)**	**16.45(4.55)**	**13.53***	1=2, 1<3, 2<3
Spelling	**13.64(6.93)**	**8.14(5.51)**	**17.73(6.17)**	**11.70***	2<1, 1=3, 2<3
K-CWST					
Word reading(C)	**94.55(22.23)**	**95.23(21.32)**	**108.14(14.85)**	**1.40**	1=2=3
Word reading(E)	**.68(.99)**	**1.05(1.84)**	**.14 (.35)**	**3.23***	1=2, 1=3, 3<2
Word reading(T)	**108.73(17.78)**	**114.64(7.12)**	**94.32(21.24)**	**6.46***	1=2, 1=3, 3<2
Color reading(C)	**57.32(31.09)**	**49.59(19.77)**	**79.32(26.69)**	**4.90***	1=2, 1=3, 2<3
Color reading(E)	**3.45(4.40)**	**5.64(9.50)**	**2.27(5.93)**	**1.41**	1=2=3
Color reading(T)	**118.86(5.33)**	**120.00(.00)**	**118.50(4.92)**	**.92**	1=2=3
Color reading(I)	**1.28(1.18)**	**1.13(.93)**	**.76 (.64)**	**.40**	1=2=3
K-MMSE					
Registration	**3.00(.00)**	**2.91(.29)**	**3.00(.00)**	**2.07**	1=2=3
Recall	**1.54(1.06)**	**1.45(1.10)**	**2.22(.87)**	**3.93***	1=2, 1<3, 2<3
SVLT					
Immediate recall	**15.32(4.48)**	**14.82(4.27)**	**18.77(4.17)**	**3.39***	1=2, 1=3, 2<3
Delayed recall	**3.77(2.14)**	**3.14(1.78)**	**5.59(2.24)**	**9.96***	1=2, 1<3, 2<3
Recognition	**18.23(2.09)**	**19.32(1.78)**	**20.05(2.19)**	**4.85***	1<2, 1<3, 2=3
RCFT					
Immediate recall	**9.93(4.51)**	**7.30(3.56)**	**13.59(5.89)**	**7.85***	2<1, 1=3, 2<3
Delayed recall	**9.82(4.53)**	**7.34(3.07)**	**13.05(5.55)**	**6.97***	2<1, 1=3, 2<3
Recognition	**18.68(2.10)**	**18.36(1.99)**	**20.00(2.39)**	**2.09**	1=2, 1=3, 2<3
Digit Span					
Forward	**5.32(1.29)**	**4.82(1.47)**	**5.55(1.26)**	**1.78**	1=2=3
Backward	**2.86(1.17)**	**3.18(.85)**	**3.64(.90)**	**1.33**	1=2=3
RCFT					
Copy	**25.63(7.10)**	**22.41(7.89)**	**28.50(5.93)**	**3.59***	2<1, 1=3, 2<3
ILP	**.77(.43)**	**.64(.49)**	**.91(.29)**	**2.08**	1=2=3
K-BNT	**37.68(9.34)**	**33.68(10.69)**	**45.54(7.79)**	**7.65***	1=2, 1<3, 2<3

(Reprinted from J Korean Neurol Assoc with permission from Korean Neurological Association (J Korean Neurol Assoc,2011))

Table 1. Neuropsychological performances of PD-MCI, svMCI, and normal control.Values shown are mean (SD). 1=PD-MCI (Parkinson disease and mild cognitive impairment), 2=svMCI (subcortical vascular mild cognitive impairment), 3=NC (normal control), K-CWST=Korean color word stroop test, SVLT: Seoul verbal learning test, RCFT=Rey complex figure test, C=correct response, E=error response, T=time per item, ILP=Interlocking Pentagon/ *p<0.05 by analysis of covariance.

2.1.3 Attention

There was no difference between normal control and both patients group in forward and backward digit span test, and no difference between patient groups.

2.1.4 Visuospatial function

In interlocking pentagon drawing of mini-mental state examination, there was no significant difference between normal control and both patient groups and neither between patient groups. On the other hand, in copy of Rey complex figure test, svMCI showed decreased performance compared to the PD-MCI group and normal controls.

2.1.5 Language

Both patient groups showed decreased performance in Boston Naming Test and there was no difference between the two patient groups.

2.1.6 Depressive mood

The PD-MCI group was more depressive than the svMCI group in Geriatric Depression Scale (Yesavage et al., 1982).

Overall, both svMCI group and PD-MCI group showed multiple domains of cognitive impairment, prominent deficit in frontal executive function and memory function. svMCI group showed severe impairment in frontal executive function, which could be attributed by both white matter and gray matter lesion, compared to the PD-MCI group which displayed severe impairment in verbal memory function. These differences in cognitive function may help to differentiate PD-MCI from svMCI and to know their pathophysiology. Interestingly, PD-MCI group also showed severe depressive mood which opens the possibility of cognitive improvement through therapy of the symptom.

2.2 Subcortical vascular dementia

2.2.1 A case presentation of subcortical vascular dementia

The patient is a 66-year-old right-handed male high school graduate. He was diagnosed with hypertension 10 years ago without but did not have drug treatment. He smoked one pack of cigarettes per day for 30 years. His mother suffered a stroke in her sixties. He is a realtor and interested in stock market. Mountain climbing with colleagues has been a longstanding hobby for several decades. He suffered a stroke-like event at 63-years old, the symptom of the event was transient left side clumsiness. The symptoms lasted for two weeks and spontaneously improved. After that event he had difficulty of subway trip because he confused finding the right entrance of familiar subway station. Moreover, sometimes he was lost on the way to his daughter's house which he was used to. The other symptom was losing money in stock market. Before the event he was quite successful in the stock exchange and earned some amount of money for several decades in stock market. The money losing in stock market was getting bigger that his wife and daughter forced him to stop stock exchange. Since three months before the first visit to memory clinic, his gait became clumsy again, on both legs, and sometimes fell on the ground during mountain climbing, which made him stop the hobby. In addition to such symptoms, mild memory deficit developed which resulted in poor management of bank account. Neuropsychological examination noted behavioral features of frontal lobe dysfunction such as aggressiveness, depressive mood, apathy, irritability and poor appetite. Magnetic resonance imaging demonstrated diffuse white matter hyperintensity prominent in frontal white matter with multiple subcortical lacunar old infarctions bilaterally on T2-weighted images. His mini-mental state examination (Folstein et al., 1975) score was 25 followed by 19 and 14 during consecutive two years. During eight years after first visit, the patient has been managed with antiplatelet agents, antihypertensive agents and atypical antipsychotics. Stroke-like symptoms did not recur but the frontal features of cognitive symptoms and gait disturbance, mild dysarthria and urinary incontinence were slowly progressing. His neuropsychological test revealed increasing deficits in multiple cognitive domains, especially in frontal executive functions. His brain MRI revealed multiple lacunar infarctions on both basal ganglia including bilateral caudate nucleus heads, globus pallidus, putamen, thalamus, and centrum semiovale on the T2 view. Diffuse white matter hyperintensities were seen, prominent in frontal lobe white matter, on the fluid attenuated inversion recovery (FLAIR) view(Figure 2). There also was frontal lobe atrophy which is severe than his age. At last contact, he became mute, urinary and fecal incontinent, bound to wheelchair and spitting to everywhere with mini-mental state examination score of 16.

This patient is a typical case of subcortical vascular dementia. He suffered several episodes of stroke-like symptoms which initiated and aggravated the cognitive symptoms and neurologic symptoms. Those symptoms improved slowly after each event, but not to the level of normal state. The pattern of cognitive decline was a stepwise pattern and antiplatelet agents and antihypertensive medication seemed to prevent further stroke-like episodes. The mini-mental state examination score showed steady state after falling to 14 during first two years which is not usual for Alzheimer's disease. However, his neurological and behavioral symptoms declined slowly to being wheelchair bound and mute.

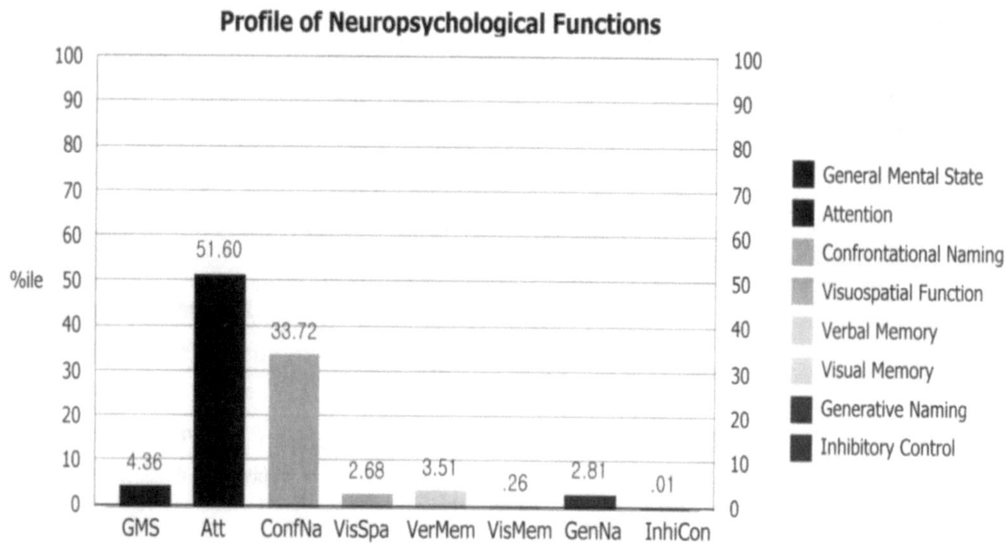

Fig. 1. Neuropsychological performance of a patient with subcortical vascular dementia. Attention and Naming were relatively preserved. Visual memory is more impaired than verbal memory. Severe impairment of frontal inhibitory function is noted.

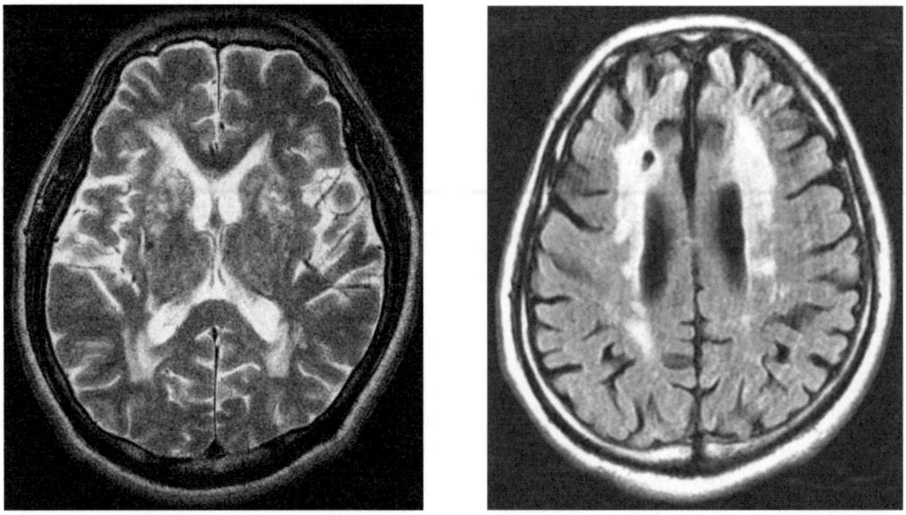

Fig. 2. Characteristic brain MRI appearances in a patient with subcortical vascular dementia. Note multiple lacunar infarctions on both basal ganglia(left, T2 image) and diffuse white matter hyperintensities(right, FLAIR image).

2.2.2 Cognitive features of subcortical vascular dementia

It has recently been proposed that patients with subcortical form of vascular dementia represent a highly prevalent and homogeneous group (Erkinjuntti et al., 2000). The primary clinical manifestation is a subcortical syndrome comprising progressive cognitive impairment with frontal features and parkinsonism poorly responsive to dopaminergic therapy (Erkinjuntti et al., 2000). Though the clinical features of subcortical vascular dementia may not show apparent stepwise deterioration, essentially the cognitive deterioration will show stepwise pattern, because of repetitive subcortical ischemic event, like lacunar infarction or other ischemic changes of subcortical structures (Loeb et al., 1992). These subcortical ischemic events including lacunar infarction frequently occur in subcortical gray matter and white matter which connect cognitive connecting pathways, like frontal-subcortical circuits, that cause frontal executive dysfunction and other cognitive deficits (Wolfe et al., 1990) and often produce a clinical syndrome like Parkinson's disease which also affect subcortical structures (Frisoni GB et al., 2002). Cerebral autosomal dominant arteriopathy with subcortical infarcts and leukoencephalopathy (CADASIL) is a genetic disorder that exhibits ischemic event as well as migraine. The cognitive symptoms of CADASIL include frontal executive dysfunction due to their subcortical involvement (Chabriat et al., 1995).

When we compare neuropsychological scores between subcortical vascular dementia and Alzheimer's disease, we can see less memory impairment and severe executive dysfunction in the patients with subcortical vascular dementia, which is exactly consistent with the results of subcortical vascular mild cognitive impairment (Table 2, Unpublished data). The two groups were matched with respect to age, sex, education, and severity of dementia (Ryu et al., 2012). The study comprised 61 patients with subcortical vascular dementia and 112 patients with Alzheimer's disease matched with respect to age, sex, education, and dementia severity. The diagnosis of dementia was based on DSM-IV criteria. The diagnosis

Neuropsychological tests (maximum possible score)	AD(n=61)	SCVD(n=112)	*P*-value* *
Attention			
Digit span			
forward	4.28(1.51)	4.36(1.32)	NS
backward	1.95(1.52)	2.00(1.23)	NS
Language & related disorders			
K-BNT (60)	24.78(12.26)	23.97(10.91)	NS
Calculation (12)	6.50(3.99)	5.95(3.51)	NS
Ideomotor limb apraxia (5)	3.78(1.37)	4.16(1.20)	NS
SVLT			
sum of three free recall (36)	8.98(4.49)	9.59(4.61)	NS
delayed recall (12)	0.58(1.42)	1.36(1.99)	≤ 0.05
recognition*	2.78(2.92)	4.28(3.12)	≤ 0.05
Visuospatial function			
RCFT (36)	13.95(10.88)	12.66(7.76)	NS
RCFT			
immediate recall (36)	3.07(3.45)	3.51(3.03)	NS
delayed recall(36)	2.20(3.16)	2.91(3.06)	NS
recognition*	2.68(2.60)	2.80(2.69)	NS
Frontal/Executive function			
COWAT			
Semantic : animal items	7.62(3.86)	7.11(3.17)	NS
Semantic : supermarket items	7.92(4.67)	7.22(3.97)	NS
phonemic: sum of three letters	7.41(8.40)	4.45(5.11)	≤ 0.05
Stroop test			
letter reading (112)	83.40(29.12)	69.06(30.46)	≤ 0.05
colour reading (112)	37.66(26.48)	29.12(22.44)	NS

Table 2. Results of neuropsychological tests of AD group and SCVD group. Values shown are mean(SD). AD, Alzheimer's disease; SCVD, subcortical vascular dementia; NS, Not-significant; K-BNT, Korean version of the Boston Naming Test; RCFT, Rey-Osterrieth Complex Figure Test; SVLT, Seoul Verbal Learning Test; COWAT, Controlled Oral Word Association Test, *true positive-false positive. * *P values by Independent T-test (Unpublished data)

of subcortical vascular dementia was also based on modified NINDS-AIREN criteria proposed by Erkinjuntti et al (2000) which requires minor neurologic symptoms and diffuse cerebral white matter lesions demonstrated on magnetic resonance imaging. The diagnosis of Alzheimer's disease was also based on NINCDS-ADRDA criteria. The Seoul Neuropsychological Screening Battery, a standardized neuropsychological battery (Kang & Na, 2003), was performed in subcortical vascular dementia and Alzheimer's disease subjects and part of the battery was performed in controls. Clinical assessments include Clinical dementia rating (CDR) (Morris, 1993), Barthel activities of daily living (B-ADL) (Mahoney & Barthel, 1965), Geriatric depression scale, and modified Hachinski ischemia scales (Rosen et al, 1980). Frontal executive dysfunction was prominent in subcortical vascular dementia in phonemic part on Controlled Oral Word Association test (COWAT) and the letter reading part on the Stroop test. Semantic COWAT and color reading on Stroop test did not show a difference between the two groups. Memory tests showed decreased performance in verbal and visuospatial memory tests for both groups. The Alzheimer's disease group showed significantly worse results on delayed recall test and recognition test in verbal learning test. Net scores of Rey complex figure test also showed worse results in Alzheimer's group but this was not significant. Ideomotor limb apraxia tests showed worse performance in Alzheimer's disease group. Boston naming test and forward and backward test of Digit span did not showed significant differences between the two groups. Interestingly, both groups showed similar grade of depressive moods on the Geriatric depression scale.

2.2.3 Strategic single infarct dementia

Strategic single infarct dementia is a type of vascular dementia and could be considered a type of subcortical vascular dementia (Bogousslavsky et al., 1988), more specifically lacunar type by the modified NINDS-AIREN criteria introduced by Erkinjuntti et al. (2000). However, it has some distinctive characteristics. The first is that a patient with strategic single infarct dementia develops dementia after one episode of stroke, not involving the cerebral cortex. Second, the lesion involved in this kind of vascular dementia is specified, like thalamus, head of caudate nucleus (Benistry et al., 2009), genu of internal capsule, posterior limb of internal capsule. Third, the cognitive deficit does not decline sharply but shows steady state as long as vascular risk factors are well controlled. Sometimes the cognitive decline aggravates even though the vascular risk factors are in good control and there is no stroke after the first episode. This could be accounted for by Wallerian degeneration of neurons as in the case of traumatic brain injury (Berker, 1996). The cognitive domains disturbed in strategic single infarct dementia depend on the location of the lesion. In the case of head of caudate nucleus infarction, dominant symptoms are frontal executive dysfunction. In thalamic infarction, there are memory symptoms as well as frontal executive dysfunction which is explained by thalamic involvement of frontal subcortical circuit and Papez circuit (Nishio et al., 2011).

2.3 Multi-infarct dementia

Multi-infarct dementia (Hachinski et al., 1974) is a common cause of dementia in patients with poorly controlled hypertension. Repeated thrombo-embolic cerebral infarctions cause typical stepwise deterioration of cognitive function as well as motor function. Main cause of cognitive dysfunction in multi-infarct dementia has been considered as large areas of cortical damage (Cummings, 1987). The cognitive features of multi-infarct dementia vary greatly with the location of strokes. The neuropsychological dysfunction may be patchy like distribution of cognitive domain which develops a dementia syndrome (Emery et al., 2000). Cerebral infarctions along the language areas frequently exhibit speaking and comprehension while infarctions of posterior cerebrum show visual agnostic symptoms and problems of reading and writing. Unless there are lesions in prefrontal lobe, there is no executive dysfunction. Therefore the cognitive symptoms of multi-infarct dementia are too various and hard to describe as one criteria of dementia.

2.4 Hemorrhagic dementia

The incidence and prevalence of hemorrhagic dementia is decreasing with better control of hypertension. However, it needs persistent attention. Multiple lobar hemorrhages, due to hypertension and/or cerebral amyloid angiopathy, may cause similar course and consequences as those of multi-infarct dementia (Itoh et al., 1993). Other causes of hemorrhagic dementia are bleeding from aneurismal rupture, amyloid angiopathy, cerebral arterio-venous malformation and chronic subdural hematoma.

3. Course of cognitive impairment in vascular dementia

The stepwise and fluctuating course of decline has been thought to result from multiple recurrent strokes in patients with vascular dementia. Each stroke may cause an acute change in the patient's level of cognitive function and may have a period of stability or partial recovery (Desmond et al., 2003). Subcortical vascular dementia typically exhibits frontal executive dysfunction and some of them show mild to moderate degree of memory impairment. When we compare memory decline of subcortical vascular dementia with Alzheimer's disease, we can notice improved recognition function than delayed recall of memory. It could be explained that memory impairments in subcortical vascular dementia were developed due to retrieval deficit, which is related to decreased attention from the frontal dysfunction compared to consolidation deficit due to direct hippocampal dysfunction of Alzheimer's disease. However this phenomenon may be dimmed when the patients with subcortical vascular dementia suffer moderate to severe degree of dementia.

In an informative study of the course of cognitive decline of multi-infarct dementia, 54% of the patients with multi-infarct dementia showed insidious onset and 50% of the patient exhibited gradually progressive course of memory decline (Fisher et al., 1990). The stereotypic cognitive decline of vascular dementia occurred in only 34% of the patients, which means two thirds of multi-infarct dementia does not show typical stepwise features. It suggests that there are many exceptions to the typical stepwise course of cognitive decline in vascular dementia and there is a large need to do brain imaging in patients with cognitive decline.

4. Summary and conclusions

There are various features of cognitive impairment in dementia syndrome. For the vascular dementia, the cognitive symptoms are mainly dependent on the ischemic or hemorrhagic lesions and severity and duration of the lesions. The course of cognitive decline may roughly match that of neurologic decline in each type of vascular dementia (Figure 3).

Figure 3 shows typical form of a time course of each type of vascular dementia. However, we should acknowledge that there could be many exceptions to such a typical form of clinical course. Moreover, a patient with multiple strokes may show cognitive characteristics of one type and later may show the other type of vascular dementia. In subcortical vascular dementia, gray matter lesions provoke more serious damage and sequela than white matter lesions. White matter lesion, mainly axonal and myelin sheath damage, may be recovered by cerebral recovering mechanism. However, gray matter damage, mainly neuronal body lesion, have little potential to be regenerated.

Multi-infarct dementia and strategic single infarct dementia was noted easily due to dramatic episode of stroke and serious neurologic deficit. However, with the introduction of skills and drugs for management of vascular risk factors such as hypertension and diabetes mellitus, the clinical importance of subcortical vascular dementia is increased. Subcortical vascular dementia shows slowly progressive cognitive decline without a dramatic stroke event such that it is difficult to distinguish subcortical vascular dementia from Alzheimer's disease. With comprehensive neuropsychological tests, predominant frontal executive dysfunction and lesser memory decline, particularly in verbal memory could be the clue to subcortical vascular dementia. Before reaching the diagnosis of vascular dementia, we should be careful to distinguish it from Alzheimer's disease because many patients with Alzheimer's disease have ischemic changes and patients with vascular dementia also may have Alzheimer's pathology in quite large proportion of such patients (Desmond et al., 2000). We could differentiate pure vascular dementia from mixed type dementia when a patient with suspected vascular dementia shows a steady cognitive state for more than several years only with management of vascular factors.

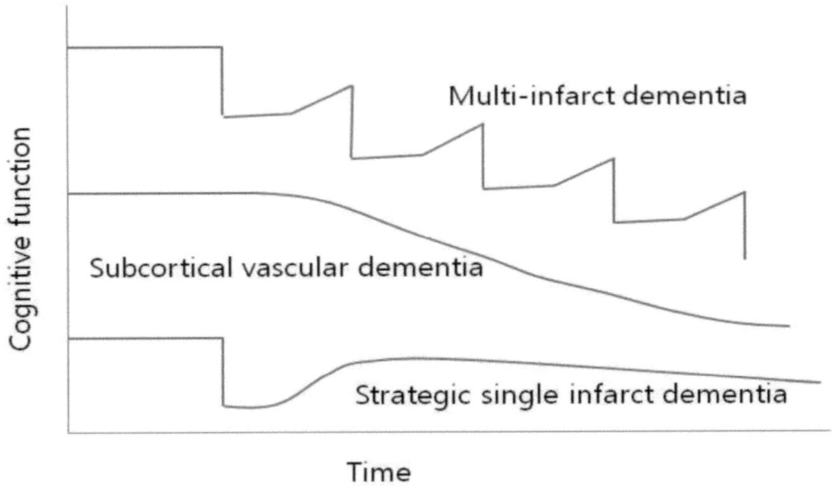

Fig. 3. Clinical course of each subtypes of vascular dementia. Multi-infarct dementia shows typical stepwise deterioration which improved a little after an acute episode until the next stroke happens. Subcortical vascular dementia shows slow, progressive decline during long periods which is similar with that of Alzheimer's disease. Strategic single infarct dementia has one serious event followed by partial recovery and steady state.

5. Acknowledgements

I wish to express my gratitude to Mrs. HJ Kim for the nice tables and figures and Ms. SY Choi, Ms. JH Kim, and Ms. JY Kim for the excellent neuropsychological tests administered to the patients. And I also thank Mr. HG Ryu for the data processing and statistical support.

6. References

American Psychiatric Association. 1994. Diagnostic and statistical manual of mental disorders : DSM-IV. Washington, D.C.: American Psychiatric Association.

Benisty S, Gouw AA, Porcher R, Madureira S, Hernandez K, Poggesi A, van der Flier WM, Van Straaten EC, Verdelho A, Ferro J, et al. 2009. Location of lacunar infarcts correlates with cognition in a sample of non-disabled subjects with age-related white-matter changes: The LADIS study. J Neurol Neurosurg Psychiatry 80(5):478-83.

Berker E. 1996. Diagnosis, physiology, pathology and rehabilitation of traumatic brain injuries. Int J Neurosci 85(3-4):195-220.

Bogousslavsky J, Regli F, Uske A. 1988. Thalamic infarcts: Clinical syndromes, etiology, and prognosis. Neurology 38(6):837-48.

Bowler JV and Hachinski V. 2003. Vascular cognitive impairment-a new concept. In: Vascular cognitive impairment. Bowler JV and Hachinski V, editors. New York, United States: Oxford University Press. 321 p.

Bowler JV, Hadar U, Wade JP. 1994. Cognition in stroke. Acta Neurol Scand 90(6):424-9.

Caviness JN, Driver-Dunckley E, Connor DJ, Sabbagh MN, Hentz JG, Noble B, Evidente VG, Shill HA, Adler CH. 2007. Defining mild cognitive impairment in parkinson's disease. Mov Disord 22(9):1272-7.

Chabriat H, Vahedi K, Iba-Zizen MT, Joutel A, Nibbio A, Nagy TG, Krebs MO, Julien J, Dubois B, Ducrocq X. 1995. Clinical spectrum of CADASIL: A study of 7 families. cerebral autosomal dominant arteriopathy with subcortical infarcts and leukoencephalopathy. Lancet 346(8980):934-9.

Chui HC, Victoroff JI, Margolin D, Jagust W, Shankle R, Katzman R. 1992. Criteria for the diagnosis of ischemic vascular dementia proposed by the state of california alzheimer's disease diagnostic and treatment centers. Neurology 42(3 Pt 1):473-80.

Cummings JL. 1987. Multi-infarct dementia: Diagnosis and management. infarctions produce 20% to 35% of severe dementia cases. Psychosomatics 28(3):117,9, 123-6.

Desmond DW. 2000. The evaluation of mood and behavior in patients with focal brain lesions. In: Behavior and mood disorders in focal brain lesions. Bogousslavsky J and Cummings JL, editors. Cambridge, England: Cambridge University Press. 21 p.

Emery VO, Gillie EX, Smith JA. 2000. Interface between vascular dementia and alzheimer syndrome. nosologic redefinition. Ann N Y Acad Sci 903:229-38.

Erkinjuntti T, Inzitari D, Pantoni L, Wallin A, Scheltens P, Rockwood K, Roman GC, Chui H, Desmond DW. 2000. Research criteria for subcortical vascular dementia in clinical trials. Journal of Neural Transmission.Supplementum 59:23-30.

Fischer P, Gatterer G, Marterer A, Simanyi M, Danielczyk W. 1990. Course characteristics in the differentiation of dementia of the alzheimer type and multi-infarct dementia. Acta Psychiatr Scand 81(6):551-3.

Folstein MF, Folstein SE, McHugh PR. 1975. "Mini-mental state". A practical method for grading the cognitive state of patients for the clinician. J Psychiatr Res 12(3):189-98.

Frisoni GB, Galluzzi S, Bresciani L, Zanetti O, Geroldi C. 2002. Mild cognitive impairment with subcortical vascular features: Clinical characteristics and outcome. J Neurol 249(10):1423-32.

Hachinski VC, Lassen NA, Marshall J. 1974. Multi-infarct dementia. A cause of mental deterioration in the elderly. Lancet 2(7874):207-10.

Itoh Y, Yamada M, Hayakawa M, Otomo E, Miyatake T. 1993. Cerebral amyloid angiopathy: A significant cause of cerebellar as well as lobar cerebral hemorrhage in the elderly. J Neurol Sci 116(2):135-41.

Kang YW and Na DL. 2003. Seoul neuropsychological screening battery. Seoul, Korea: Human Brain Research & Consulting Co.

Kim JH, Jin YS, Chang MS, Choi SY, Kwon OD. 2011. Neuropsychological characteristics of mild cognitibe impairment in parkinson's disease and subcortical vascular mild cognitive impairment. J Korean Neurol Assoc 29:311-6.

Kittner B, De Deyn PP, Erkinjuntti T. 2000. Investigating the natural course and treatment of vascular dementia and alzheimer's disease. parallel study populations in two randomized, placebo-controlled trials. Ann N Y Acad Sci 903:535-41.

Loeb C, Gandolfo C, Croce R, Conti M. 1992. Dementia associated with lacunar infarction. Stroke 23(9):1225-9.

Mahoney FI and Barthel DW. 1965. Functional evaluation: The barthel index. Md State Med J 14:61-5.

McKhann G, Drachman D, Folstein M, Katzman R, Price D, Stadlan EM. 1984. Clinical diagnosis of alzheimer's disease: Report of the NINCDS-ADRDA work group under the auspices of department of health and human services task force on alzheimer's disease. Neurology 34(7):939-44.

McKinlay A, Grace RC, Dalrymple-Alford JC, Roger D. 2009. Cognitive characteristics associated with mild cognitive impairment in parkinson's disease. Dement Geriatr Cogn Disord 28(2):121-9.

Morris JC. 1993. The clinical dementia rating (CDR): Current version and scoring rules. Neurology 43(11):2412-4.

Nishio Y, Hashimoto M, Ishii K, Mori E. 2011. Neuroanatomy of a neurobehavioral disturbance in the left anterior thalamic infarction. J Neurol Neurosurg Psychiatry .

Petersen RC, Smith GE, Waring SC, Ivnik RJ, Tangalos EG, Kokmen E. 1999. Mild cognitive impairment: Clinical characterization and outcome. Arch Neurol 56(3):303-8.

Roman GC, Erkinjuntti T, Wallin A, Pantoni L, Chui HC. 2002. Subcortical ischaemic vascular dementia. Lancet Neurol 1(7):426-36.

Rosen WG, Terry RD, Fuld PA, Katzman R, Peck A. 1980. Pathological verification of ischemic score in differentiation of dementias. Ann Neurol 7(5):486-8.

Ryu HG, Youn SW, Kwon OD. 2012. Lack of association between apolipoprotein E polymorphism with age at onset of subcortical vascular dementia. Dement Geriatr Cogn Disord Extra 2:1-9.

Tatemichi TK, Desmond DW, Mayeux R, Paik M, Stern Y, Sano M, Remien RH, Williams JB, Mohr JP, Hauser WA. 1992. Dementia after stroke: Baseline frequency, risks, and clinical features in a hospitalized cohort. Neurology 42(6):1185-93.

Wolfe N, Linn R, Babikian VL, Knoefel JE, Albert ML. 1990. Frontal systems impairment following multiple lacunar infarcts. Arch Neurol 47(2):129-32.

Yesavage JA, Brink TL, Rose TL, Lum O, Huang V, Adey M, Leirer VO. 1982. Development and validation of a geriatric depression screening scale: A preliminary report. J Psychiatr Res 17(1):37-49.

[25] Ghirardello S, Hopper N, Albanese A, Maghnie M. Diabetes insipidus in craniopharyngioma: postoperative management of water and electrolyte disorders. J Pediatr Endocrinol Metab. 2006 Apr;19 Suppl 1:413-21.

[26] Haraguchi K, Morimoto S, Tanooka A, Inoue M, Yoshida Y. [Craniopharyngioma presenting a symptom of pituitary apoplexy and hyponatremia: a case report]. No Shinkei Geka. 2000 Dec;28(12):1111-5.

[27] Tao Y, Lian D, Hui-Juan Z, Hui P, Zi-Meng J. Value of brain magnetic resonance imaging and tumor markers in the diagnosis and treatment of intracranial germinoma in children. Zhongguo Yi Xue Ke Xue Yuan Xue Bao. 2011 Apr;33(2):111-5.

[28] Kreutz J, Rausin L, Weerts E, Tebache M, Born J, Hoyoux C. Intracranial germ cell tumor. JBR-BTR. 2010 Jul-Aug;93(4):196-7.

[29] Kim YS, Kang SG, Kim YO. Pituitary teratoma presenting as central diabetes insipidus with a normal MRI finding. Yonsei Med J. 2010 Mar 1;51(2):293-4.

[30] Sandow BA, Dory CE, Aguiar MA, Abuhamad AZ. Best cases from the AFIP: congenital intracranial teratoma. Radiographics. 2004 Jul-Aug;24(4):1165-70.

[31] Carpinteri R, Patelli I, Casanueva FF, Giustina A. Pituitary tumours: inflammatory and granulomatous expansive lesions of the pituitary. Best Pract Res Clin Endocrinol Metab. 2009 Oct;23(5):639-50.

[32] Rosenzweig KE, Arceci RJ, Tarbell NJ. Diabetes insipidus secondary to Langerhans' cell histiocytosis: is radiation therapy indicated? Med Pediatr Oncol. 1997 Jul;29(1):36-40.

[33] Hermet M, Delévaux I, Trouillier S, André M, Chazal J, Aumaître O. [Pituitary metastasis presenting as diabetes insipidus: a report of four cases and literature review]. Rev Med Interne. 2009 May;30(5):425-9.

[34] Martinez JR, Grantham JJ. Polycystic kidney disease: etiology, pathogenesis, and treatment. Dis Mon. 1995 Nov;41(11):693-765.

[35] Onuigbo MA, Skalski J. Newly symptomatic central diabetes insipidus in ESRD with adult polycystic kidney disease following intracranial hemorrhage: the first reported case. Med Sci Monit. 2010 Feb 26;16(3):CS29-32.

[36] Grünfeld JP, Rossier BC. Lithium nephrotoxicity revisited. Nat Rev Nephrol. 2009 May;5(5):270-6.

[37] Jung DC, Kim SH, Jung SI, Hwang SI, Kim SH. Renal papillary necrosis: review and comparison of findings at multi-detector row CT and intravenous urography. Radiographics. 2006 Nov-Dec;26(6):1827-36.

[38] Köhler H, Weber M, Wandel E, Schild HH. [The analgesic-damaged kidney. Importance of the imaging procedure]. Dtsch Med Wochenschr. 1987 Aug 28;112(35):1347-52.

[39] Smith EA. Pyelonephritis, renal scarring, and reflux nephropathy: a pediatric urologist's perspective. Pediatr Radiol. 2008 Jan;38 Suppl 1:S76-82.

[40] Eggli DF, Tulchinsky M. Scintigraphic evaluation of pediatric urinary tract infection. Semin Nucl Med. 1993 Jul;23(3):199-218.

[41] Chang SL, Caruso TJ, Shortliffe LD. Magnetic resonance imaging detected renal volume reduction in refluxing and nonrefluxing kidneys. J Urol. 2007 Dec;178(6):2550-4.

[42] Lee VW, Skinner M, Cohen AS, Ngai S, Peng TT. Renal amyloidosis. Evaluation by gallium imaging. Clin Nucl Med. 1986 Sep;11(9):642-6.

[43] Hachulla E, Maulin L, Deveaux M, Facon T, Blétry O, Vanhille P, Wechsler B, Godeau P, Levesque H, Hatron PY, Huglo D, Devulder B, Marchandise X. Prospective and serial study of primary amyloidosis with serum amyloid P component scintigraphy: from diagnosis to prognosis. Am J Med. 1996 Jul;101(1):77-87.
[44] Kim SH, Han JK, Lee KH, Won HJ, Kim KW, Kim JS, Park CH, Choi BI. Abdominal amyloidosis: spectrum of radiological findings. Clin Radiol. 2003 Aug;58(8):610-20.
[45] Dupas B, Buzelin MF, Karam G, Vasse N, Meflah K, Bach-Gansmo T. Contrast-enhanced MR imaging of experimental acute tubular necrosis. Acta Radiol. 2001 Jan;42(1):74-9.
[46] Platt JF, Rubin JM, Ellis JH. Acute renal failure: possible role of duplex Doppler US in distinction between acute prerenal failure and acute tubular necrosis. Radiology. 1991 May;179(2):419-23.

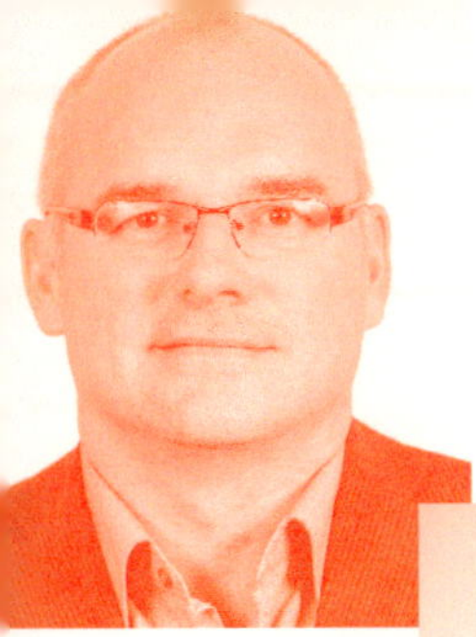
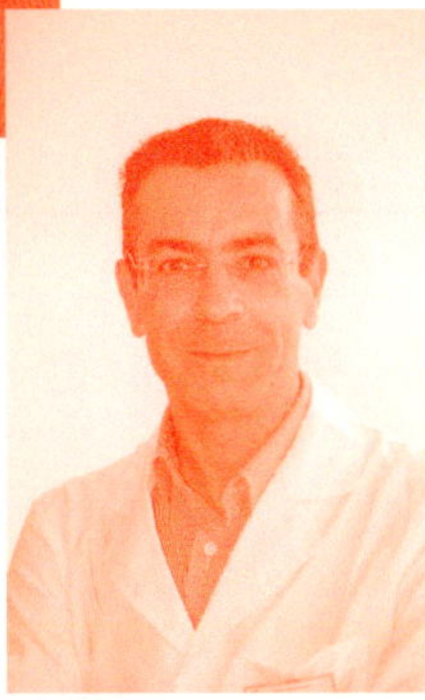
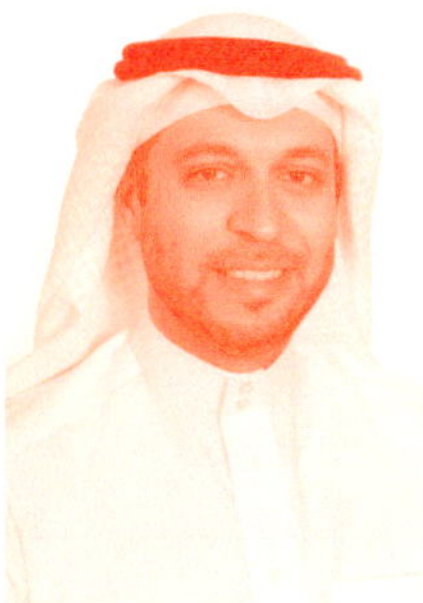
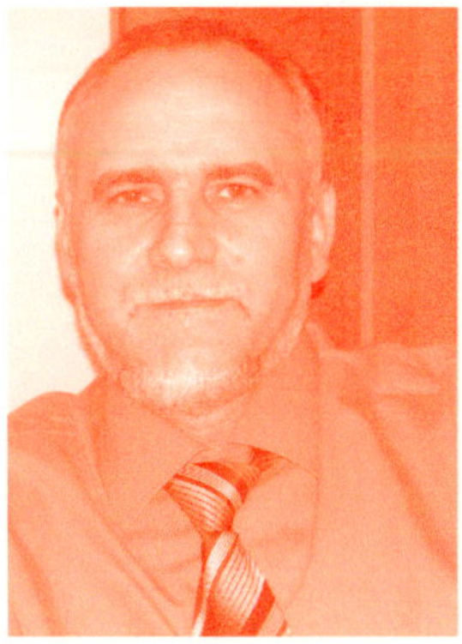
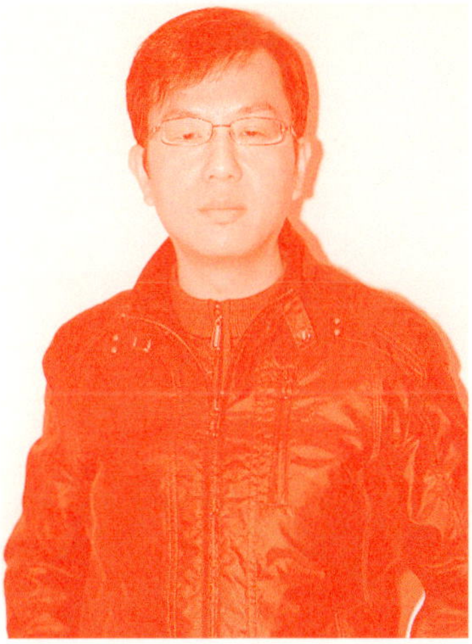
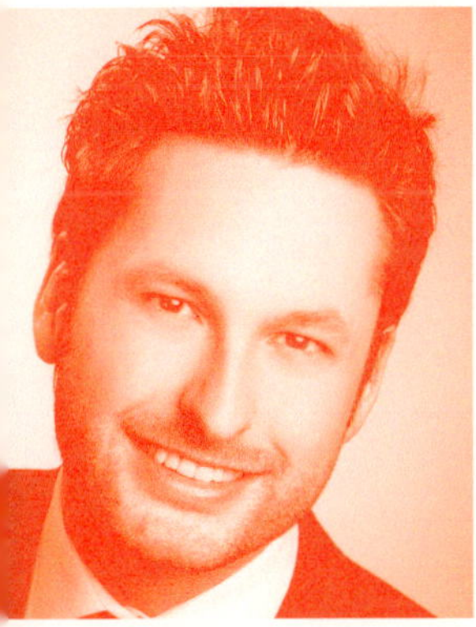
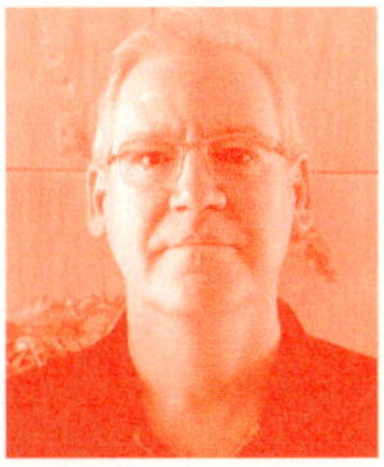

IntechOpen

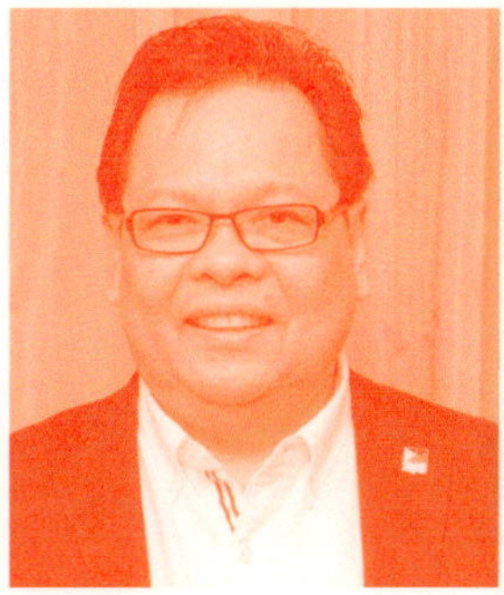
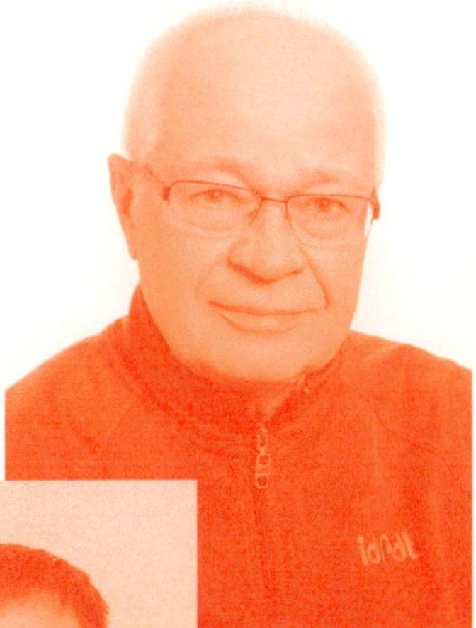
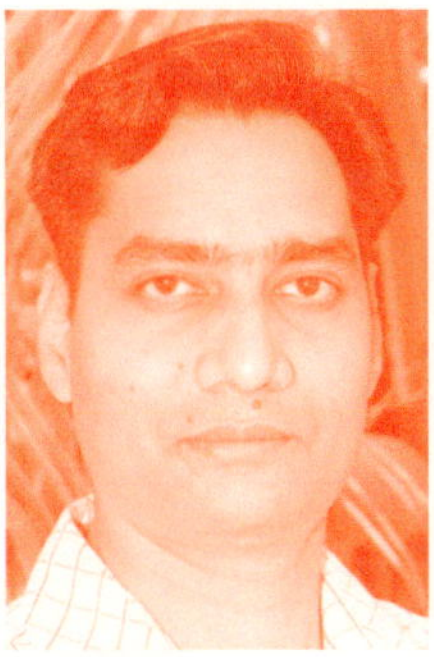
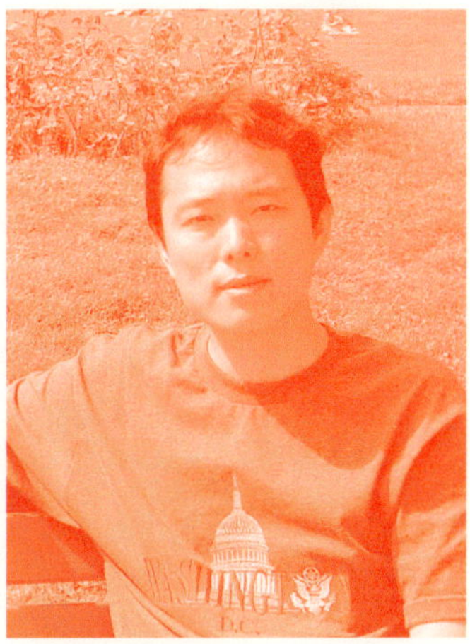
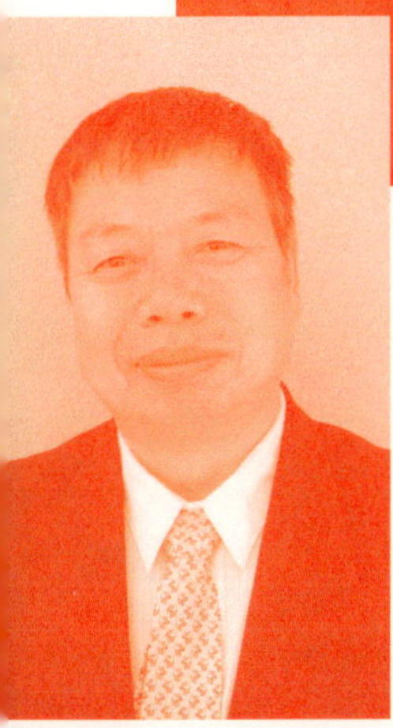
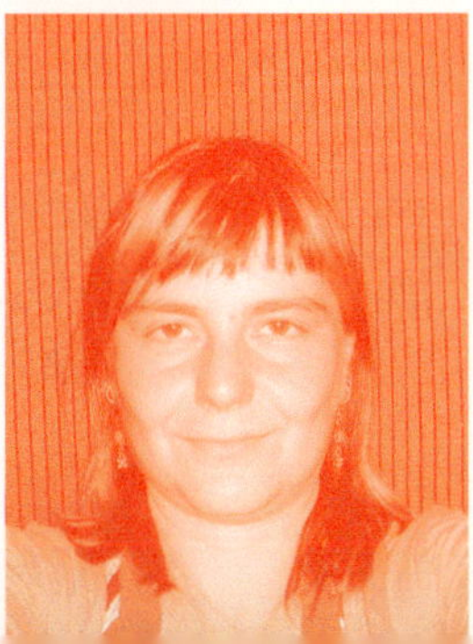

Leishmaniasis - General Aspects of a Stigmatized Disease

Edited by Leonardo de Azevedo Calderon

Published in London, United Kingdom